THE

NEURO CARE

MANUAL

(A guide to neurology for nurses and family carers)

*Nursing **p**eople who have advanced
Parkinson's disease, **P**ick's disease
Huntington's disease
&
Alzheimer's disease
Lewy Body dementia
Multi infarct dementia, **M**ultiple Sclerosis, **M**otor
Neurone disease &
Other
Neurological
Disorders including
Stroke*

STEVE SMITH

HEALTH 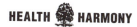 HARMONY

An imprint of

B. Jain Publishers (P) Ltd.

An ISO 9001 : 2000 Certified Company
USA — Europe — India

THE NEURO CARE MANUAL

First Edition: 2011
1st Impression: 2011

Published by Kuldeep Jain for

HEALTH 🌳 **HARMONY**
An imprint of
B. JAIN PUBLISHERS (P) LTD.
An ISO 9001 : 2000 Certified Company
1921/10, Chuna Mandi, Paharganj, New Delhi 110 055 (INDIA)
Tel.: +91-11-4567 1000 • Fax: +91-11-4567 1010
Email: info@bjain.com • Website: www.bjain.com

Printed in India by

ISBN: 978-81-319-0844-0

The book is dedicated to my dear Mum, Rene, who after tireless and loving and joyful dedication to the family, the community and the world, is courageously facing challenges that are part of the subject matter of this book .

Foreword

'Language is an inventory of human experience.'

\- L.W. Lockhart

I am a nurse. I care for patients. Together with physicians and physiotherapists, occupational therapists and speech therapists, nutritionalists and social workers, we all band together to care for patients and their families. And while some may pride themselves on being able to communicate clearly to those we care for, the fact remains that we sometimes fall short. Could the language we speak sometimes be the reason? As L.W. Lockhart reminds us, the language we use emanates from our experiences. So how do we reconcile our career-speak to caring-speak?

Steve Smith, a dear and insightful friend of mine since many years, has maintained that we as care givers engage with families with the best of intentions, but our dialogue is different. It is as if we are attempting to connect to the family yet that linkage is not always achieved. This book provides a bridge for professionals to reach the destination of relating to the family. He has been able to distill the essence of professional language to 'people-speak' in order to help the inventory of the human experience be more readily understood by all the parties.

This book is written in a very simple language, certainly not to undermine the professional language we have grown accustomed to and use in our everyday professional conversations. Rather to add to our armentarium of understanding the effects of neurodegenerative disorders and enhancing our communication with those that love the patients afflicted with these diseases the most—their loved ones. This is a book that can and should, be used by any professional anywhere in the world as well as by family caregivers. I commend Steve for his dedication to patients and their families. He has made me a better nurse.

Virginia Prendergast, RN, MSN, CNRN
President
World Federation of Neuroscience Nurses

Preface

This book is about the challenge of nursing people with a degenerative brain disease. The term 'nursing' is used in a broad sense referring primarily to qualified nurses; but also to health care assistants and to spouses, family members, friends or neighbours or others who in some way provide informal care.

I know that the risk here is trying to produce a text that can be read by both qualified nurses and informal caregivers, among whom there will be a very wide range of relevant prior understanding, is that of patronising those with a good working knowledge, while baffling and overloading those just wanting to have some general ideas about the conditions, how they affect people and some tips about ways of handling situations. One possible option would have been to write two separate books.

The reason I want to reach both the categories of readers through one book is because we have to work together as a team if we wish to be effective. We shouldn't speak different languages. Why shouldn't nurses and other health professionals be reminded to use language others can access? And why shouldn't family members affected by neurological disease and expected to work with nurses be helped to understand some terminology that professionals use like anatomy and physiology and pathophysiology that professionals find helpful to know about and discuss among themselves?

I do hope this text will enable people at both ends and all along this spectrum to talk together more. And that talking together on a shared level, aids working together for shared aims and outcomes.

The names and in many cases other personal identifying factors of people referred to throughout the book, other than authors and experts cited are changed to protect confidentiality.

Steve Smith

Acknowledgements

My thanks to the publishers, for their patient support and encouragement and in particular Dr Geeta Rani Arora. Thanks also to those who gave comments on the manuscript: Deborah Chinman, Norfolk, England; and Trese McGrath of Redhill Surrey UK and Jo McLellan of Addiscombe, UK; all experts. I take full responsibility for any slips, but comments were very helpful and gratefully received. For more general support I am grateful to Cath Stanley, Head of Care Services- England and Wales, Huntington's Disease Association; and Marie, Gillian, John, Isobel, of the Scottish Huntington's Association; The Florence Nightingale Foundation for two scholarships, provided with invaluable advice and support. Also I thank them for the privilege and experience of serving as a Nightingale Scholar on the Executive Committee for the past four years. To Jimmy Pollard, Massachusetts, USA, and Carol Moskowitz, New York USA, Bert and Judy Chapman great teachers that I hope I haven't let down. The World Federation of Neuroscience Nurses have given me enormous ongoing support, with special thanks to Virginia, President, and to JD, Chief Executive, and to Tess (and Jim), Cindy, and Peter (of course), and to Vicky, Chair of the Scientific Programme Committee. Also to friends at the Barrow Neurological institute, Phoenix, Arizona. My friends and colleagues at the University of East Anglia, School of Nursing and Midwifery, Faculty of Health. And I owe huge thanks to my ever supportive wife, Sioux, and to all my family especially the latest additions, Elizabeth, Reuben Apollo, and Saul Lennon. Mostly however, I owe my thanks to the many people affected by neurological disease, directly or as family members, that I have come to know through my work and research activity. The courage and optimism I have encountered through them is truly inspirational. It is a privilege to have got to know them, thank you.

Publisher's Note

Neurological diseases in general and Alzheimer's disease in particular are in a category which are still not curable by the medical field today. But human nature is such that it will not fall prey to these conditions and it will devise ways to how one can survive and live with these conditions in the best possible ways.

The reason for the mystery of such diseases is the complex nature of the nervous system. There are millions of neurons in our body which are working each and every second to transmit different kinds of signals, many of which go unnoticed by us. This is evident when we remove the hand in response to a pin prick before we realize it has happened. The nervous system works like a network of interacting electrical connections. Even when you are reading this page, there are thousands of neurons working to help you concentrate, fix that vision and help understand what you have seen on paper and interpret it.

To know how to manage and take care of such patients we need to understand the nature of disease in and out. Smith has exactly done this by explaining all aspects of disease in the beginning and then has gone to finer details of the management. He says that managing a person suffering from a degenerative disease is not one person's job but a collective effort from both the qualified nurses and the caregivers. The book is therefore addressed to both the nurses and the caregivers.

The book talks about the normal structure and functions of the brain and further explains the changes that happen in different parts of the brain, the physical changes which happen due to the effects of each of such disease and the psychological and emotional aspects of it, and the treatment offered by conventional medicine. The author discusses other aspects which are very important in managing of such cases like financial aspects, emotional aspects, caring at home, safety aspects, communication, doing daily chores etc.

The book is like an emotional journey to managing Alzheimer's and all such neurological disorders with an in depth study on all practical aspects which need to be looked into.

Kuldeep Jain
C.E.O., B. Jain Publishers (P) Ltd.

Contents

INTRODUCTION

Andrew, Tim and Mary

Mary had lived at our nursing home for several years since her husband Andrew and son Tim reluctantly admitted to support workers that they just could no longer manage caring for her. Mary had been given a 'probable' diagnosis of Alzheimer's disease a couple of years prior to her nursing home admission, after becoming increasingly forgetful and socially withdrawn.

Andrew and Tim had in fact noticed a worrying change in Mary's presentation and behaviour for longer than that-before she unexpectedly gave up her teaching career. She just wasn't her old self. She was less happy and outgoing; full of excuses to avoid going out with friends or having them around and a little short tempered when something didn't go her way. It really wasn't like the Mary whom Andrew had married, and whom young Tim, now 20, had been used to and loved.

The neurologist told Mary and Andrew the diagnosis. He explained that he could only say 'probable' because a definitive diagnosis wouldn't be made until brain tissue would be analysed after death. But as far as they were concerned, it was confirmed. To their surprise the news brought them a strange sense of relief. It wasn't a shock, Andrew told me, because they both knew something awful was going on, and it just felt a bit better to be told what it was. Andrew was 51 and Mary was 49.

During good days, Mary was insightful about her condition and expressed a lot of concern for Andrew and Tim. They should move on with life. Andrew was a busy solicitor. Tim had finished an electrician's apprenticeship and had at last found a nice steady girlfriend. Mary was keen it should all carry on. She was keen to stay at home while she was safe enough to be left in the home while they went about their day, but often emphasised that the moment she was causing them to take time from work, she should go into care. Mary had visited a number of homes and chosen the one where she felt she would be happy to spend her last years.

During the days when Mary was not keeping well she didn't have this insight. She chastised the men in the house for things that went wrong. She seemed cold and unconcerned about almost all other things other than her immediate needs. She left hot plates burning, bath and sink taps running, flooding the house. Andrew did begin taking time off from his work to keep an eye on Mary, and despite what Mary said on the better days, he intended to support her at home until the end. It was her home. He loved her and could not accept her going into care. Anyway, he'd seen the other residents where Mary planned to go, and they seemed in a much worse condition than Mary. She just wouldn't fit!

But as time progressed, the good days were increasingly outnumbered by the bad ones, and Mary's condition became worse. She began to wander. She would leave the house to go shopping nearby, and Andrew would find her hours later, miles away from the shops unable to explain where she was heading. She would laugh inappropriately or burst into tears, and then, chat as though nothing untoward had happened!

Andrew woke up one night and realised that he was alone. He discovered that the front door was open and Mary was not in the house. He found her during the following morning on a park bench in her nightwear. He was afraid of what might happen next. Worse, he found that he was losing patience. He was angry at himself because he knew Mary couldn't help her condition. But he had clenched his fist a couple of times when she swore at him and demanded his help unreasonably. She was critical of all his efforts to help her.

Our nursing home was secure. It was possible to walk in and out of the big house, into large garden areas surrounded by a circular wall. Mary could wander freely within limits that she seemed unaware of and come to no harm. Kitchens were safely inaccessible, and the many large rooms meant that Mary could occupy spaces without getting into many confrontational situations, no one having to ask her to turn around, or mind the way, the kinds of situations that seemed to trigger her hostile behaviour at home. So the pleasant side of Mary seemed to return. Things generally went her way, and she was calm and content.

Andrew and Tim visited every Saturday. The cheerfulness and serenity in Mary evoked mixed feelings. Of course they were happy that she was fine and accepted that the decision to admit her was the right one. But a sense of failure was hard to beat off despite assurances. They worried about questions such as 'how come they couldn't manage to make her this happy and content in her own home?' So, whatever happened, they would always maintain the Saturday visits and sometimes midweek also. Mary's deterioration was gradual over several years. The staff and I got to know Andrew and Tim pretty well, and it happened that they tended to spend much more time speaking to us than with Mary. That's because she would smile and nod at them when they arrived, as she did to all visitors and staff coming through the door, but then she ignored them by walking off.

One Saturday Tim didn't come. Andrew explained he was tied up at work. Each week from then on, Andrew came alone, always with a tale of something unexpected cropping up for Tim. Then, Andrew and Tim did both come and they asked to see me, in a quiet room. 'Steve', Andrew said, with his head down, 'I just can't come any more and neither can Tim'. 'I don't think Mary would want us to'. Before I could think of something helpful to say, Andrew continued, 'As far as I'm concerned, Mary, whom I married and will always love, died some time ago. She was waning for a long time, but she was in there. But she isn't now. I'm not sure when exactly it happened, but I've known for some time that the body walking about is not Mary. It's a shell that she used to live in'

Tim said nothing. Andrew carried on, 'Visiting her and seeing her in here, incapacitated was always painful. It tears me apart from within every time...... We can barely speak in the car. But we vowed to do it until she died, because we can't just abandon her, and we love her. But she did die. There's no person in that head. I've thought about it. Physically her brain keeps her lungs breathing and her heart pumping blood, and so she can walk around and make gestures that are just reactions to a stimulus. So she smiles. The same smile to me, to you, to the plumber. She has no idea who Tim and I are. We just held her hands and said goodbye, but she didn't recognise us. The brain is working, but there's nobody inside it. She's gone, we must accept it. Unless you can tell me I'm wrong, Steve, and that she is in there. If you can't tell me that, we will not come back. There's just no point in enduring so much pain to visit someone who has no idea who we are once we go.'

I can't remember what I said to them. I do hope it was sufficiently sensitive and empathetic. I doubt that it was, because it must have come from the top of my head, and even now, sitting quietly and reflecting on the scenario, I struggle to think of something adequate.

Where am I?

Andrew really stumped me with his question. Was Mary still in that head of hers? Can a body and brain really function without the person being in there? What is the person then... something separate from the body that lives in it... that can die while the body is still alive? I'd never really thought about it. I think most of us can get through life without having to consider it. We may have religious or other philosophical beliefs. I'm not so sure that's quite the same as being confronted with this question. I guess Andrew never thought about it- until he was faced with it. If Mary is walking around in the nursing home, he would feel compelled to keep visiting. If she had died and was no longer present, he would draw a close to the visits in good conscience.

Seeing the Person

While it is important to understand the way that some people with a disease affecting the brain may feel they are losing their sense of who they are, and some loved ones may also sense the loss, professional nurses cannot afford to lose sight of the person. It is essential to see the person beyond the deteriorating body, impaired memory and concentration and poorly controlled movement and posture. Jimmy Pollard writes about caring for people with Huntington's disease in 'Hurry up and wait' (2008). He talks about the features of this condition- movement disorder, cognitive decline and psychiatric problems as the 'Huntington's disguise'. These 'masks' prevent us from seeing the person, until we manage to look beneath what is superficial.

We can (we should) understand why an individual maybe lost to themselves and to those who love them, but we should strive to see the person.

We should work to help re-construct the aspects of the personality that have become fragmented. Depending on the diagnosis, these might control the movement and posture, mannerisms, organisation of thinking, verbal and non-verbal communication, capacity to pay attention, to store memories and to retrieve them, or any of the numerous other functions that the brain plays a role in.

If personality is closely tied to memories, experiences, our past life, our likes and dislikes, emotions and so on, then nurses working at restoring the person to some extent, need to know and familiarise themselves with as much about these aspects of the person as is possible. I know that if I was diagnosed with a disease affecting my brain, I would like nurses caring for me to see my photo albums and any video clips of me at work, teaching student nurses; at Wimbledon, cheering on Andy Murray, playing with my grandchildren, playing the guitar or walking in the hills with my wife, Sioux.

I hope they wouldn't only see a patient with unreasonable behaviour, poor co-ordination and swallowing problems. They would try to see 'me'.

Restoring the Past isn't Possible

When I suggest that we should work to try and restore the person, or the personality, I don't mean try to get things back to the way they were. This isn't going to happen, I hate to say. An enormous challenge for families is to accept this. The conditions we are dealing with in this book are 'progressive' or 'degenerative'. Hopefully science will in future find a way to halt this process of deterioration but currently, and for the foreseeable future, it can't be done.

So what do I mean then? I'm going to assume you're an adult reading this. Are you the same person you were when you were 5 or 15? Yes, in a way, but not in aspects. There's an unbroken continuity. Barely a cell is left that was part of your body when you were a child. It's all been renewed. You don't think the way you used to and I'll bet you don't believe some of the things you did then, and you see the world differently now. What do you remember of being that age? Some details perhaps, and some facts. One or two memorable moments? But mostly, those days have gone, it's a blur. You've moved on. More than that, you are a different person to the one who is now only a memory. In fact, the memory, brief and patchy though it is, is not the same as that person was in reality anyway. It's a memory that makes sense in an adult mind.

Just, as the saying goes, a person can't stand in the same river twice, you will never again have the same mind... not if the mind is made up of your memories and experiences, and personality, because these are constantly changing and being renewed with newer experiences, fuzzier memories and newer memories, and a different, older personality. I recently enjoyed two pints of Guiness outside the Royal Festival Hall, just watching the River Thames in London. When I put down the second empty glass, none of the water I'd been looking at when I started the first was still there, but I knew it was still the River Thames... not the same one though.

The child and the adolescent that you once were are gone; they no longer exist. If you can accept and feel comfortable with who you are now, then the passing of the child and the adolescent isn't such a problem. Although they've passed, they will always be part of who you are. It is still you after all. Even though you can't recall what you did or said on most of those days.

That's what I mean about restoring the person. The loss of the adult who existed before the onset of a degenerative neurological condition is a tragedy, and very hard to come to terms with for the person, the family or their close friends. There is a feeling that the whole person is lost! But that doesn't have to be. Although, life will never be the same, and the person has moved on from the life they knew, there is still a continuity. What we can help to restore is self esteem, honour, self respect, dignity, contentment, and acceptance of the new phase of life. These things make up the person. The past, although mostly forgotten in many cases (not all degenerative neurological conditions involve losing memory) is never-the-less part of who the person is.

If the person cannot recall anything at all of their past, it still helps that we know something about it. Knowing who he or she has been, helps us understand who he or she is now, and being understood and accepted for who you are adds to self esteem and dignity.

If we can help to restore these aspects of a personality, we are doing a good job. The person will have moved on, but will be intact. Who we are does not depend on whether we can do the things we used to or remember them. Who we are depends on our levels of those very attributes: dignity, self respect, contentment and so on. 'Who we are' is enhanced by the extent to which others around us can accept our changes, and help us maintain those qualities.

Plasticity

Having said that we can't halt the progression of a degenerative neurological disease, it's not all hopeless by any means. There is a lot we can do to stimulate the functioning of the brain, even when its cells are dying off at an alarming rate. The many intriguing and uplifting books by Baroness Susan Greenfield (for example, 'ID:

The Quest for Identity in the 21st Century' (2008); The Private life of the Brain (2000); The Human Brain: A Guided Tour (1998); testify so well to what is called the brain's 'plasticity'. The word means 'ability to be moulded'. We hear so much about genes these days, and how they dictate the shape of our biological make-up, including the shape of our brains and the way they work and make us think and behave. Genes do definitely play a big part in our make-up, but they don't determine who we are, how we think and what we do. They are a factor, an important one, but they are not as in charge as we often might feel led to believe.

The environment around us, our life experiences, and interactions with those around us are certainly as important in determining how the components of our brains connect up and work, and how we think and behave. And practice improves the brain just like limbering up in the gym builds up the muscles in the arms and legs and the rest of the body. In 1999, Dr Eleanor McGuire led a famous study at the Wellcome Department of Cognitive Neurology at the University College London, analysing the brains of 16 London taxi drivers, and 50 other members of the general public (McGuire et al 1999). London 'cabbies' have to learn every street in London and are tested on their knowledge of routes to and from various locations without recourse to any notes or maps. The 'hippocampus' in the cabbie's brains were larger than those in the comparison group. So regardless of the way genetics may have influenced their brain sizes, this was changed by their activity in learning the streets of London (I don't mean the song 'Streets of London' by Ralph McTell, but that may help too).

Susan Greenfield makes this point and also cites a study by Van Dellen et al (2000). Huntington's disease, as we will see further on, is unusual in the sense that for most of the degenerative brain disorders we will consider, there are many factors that seem to play important parts in how they develop. But Huntington's disease (HD) is what we tend to call a 'single-gene' disorder. Because of a problem with one gene, the brain will deteriorate to an extent that is easily shown on a brain scan. So, you could be tempted to think that there is nothing that can be done to slow the onslaught; because each person affected by HD is an individual, and so is the way the disease seems to impact. It is not easy to make comparisons and show that one lifestyle helped slow the disease more than another lifestyle. If a man (or lady) with HD exercises a lot, and the disease seems to progress slowly, we can't be sure whether in that person there would have been a difference if he or she hadn't exercised.

And so, the researchers (Van Dellen et al) studied mice who had been genetically manipulated to have a condition that mimics HD in humans. The mice were all closely matched in every way except that some were placed into a 'dull' environment, without much to do, and some were put into a 'stimulating' environment with wheels and ladders etc to play with. The symptoms of HD in the 'stimulated' mice began later in life than in the other mice, and there was measurably less loss of the brain volume in the stimulated mice over time.

What is my point? Well, maybe we can't change the fact that someone has a degenerative neurological diagnosis. We can't turn the clock back and have the person the way they were. But we are not powerless. By making the environment enriched and stimulating, encouraging mental activity and fostering interaction with others, interests in hobbies, maybe sport, the news, puzzles, trips down memory lane aided by photographs, laughter and subtle humour, practising walking and other exercise as able and as recommended by the physician and therapists, we can help to greatly reduce the way the disease is able to disrupt enjoyment of and satisfaction with life, even in advanced stages.

PART A
THE NUTS & BOLTS

The Anatomy and Physiology of the Nervous System

Health Warning: As I repeat, a bit further on, being able to care well for a person with a neurological condition doesn't depend on you being knowledgeable about the anatomy and physiology of the nervous system. It would be fine to skip this chapter, or dip into parts that look manageable, or maybe come back to certain sections if and when they seem relevant to problems you are dealing with. Some people are happy to give good care without wanting to know any of this. Others find it very helpful to think about what it is that maybe going wrong. It can help some people to stay patient with a person who is acting strangely or unreasonably, if they can picture why this might be happening. So, read the chapter if you find it helpful, and don't worry if you need to skip part or all of if.

It is easier to think about the nervous system if we divide it into parts, so long as we keep in mind that no such divisions really exist it is a very integrated dynamic system. Traditionally, it has been divided both structurally and functionally.

The structural division is between the central nervous system (CNS) and the peripheral nervous system (PNS). The CNS includes the brain and spinal cord, and the PNS includes everything else- that is, the nerves that branch from the CNS and convey impulses to and from muscles and organs all over the body.

Functionally, there is the Somatic system (Soma means body) that you control and the Autonomic Nervous System (ANS) that controls you, making your heart beat, making you breathe, sweat, shiver, digest your food, and control your blood pressure, etc, without you having to think about it. In a simplistic way, that's the nervous system all divided up, making it manageable to think about.

Cells

There are two main types of cells in the nervous system. Those that conduct electrical impulses are called neurons. The rest are known as neuroglia, or glial cells. What do I mean by 'cells'? Well, these are the basic units in biology, and were given that name by an Austrian monk- Gregor Mendel (1822-1888) who studied sweet peas (who else would have time for that?) and became the 'father of genetics'. He likened the basic biological units and their relationship to the whole body, to the small rooms where the monks slept and their relationship to the monastery. Their little rooms were called cells.

The Glial cells (glia means glue) support and hold the rest of the nervous system in place, protect it, clean up impurities and any invading nasty cells that shouldn't be there. They have a role in regulating fluid around the nervous system too. So they're very important and there are many more of them than Neurons.

The neurons do the job of sending signals.

I mentioned that Mendel is credited with naming the basic biological unit as a 'cell'. Well, the nerve cell, or neuron, was identified through the work of two brilliant people: Camillo Golgi (Spanish, 1843-1926), and Ramón y Cajal (Italian, 1852-1934). Golgi dyed brain tissue with a silver chromate solution (a browny-red chemical mixture that was involved in early photography) and found that only a fairly small number of neurons became darkly stained. He concluded that nervous tissue was made up of a continuous web of cells.

But Cajal tried this and came up with a different way in which the cells are organised and behave. He suggested that the nervous system consists of billions of separate, individual neurons that communicate with each other across gaps, later named 'synapses', rather than form a web. The way electrical activity fires across these gaps had partly been explained in Golgi's theory. So in 1906 these two clever scientists shared the Nobel Prize in Physiology and Medicine.

Between them, all that time ago, they left us pretty much with the understanding that we have today of how neurons look and work.

The cell body of a neuron is rather like that of the typical body cells found in tissues such as skin, bone, muscle and the organs. What makes neurons different to the other cells are the long fibres extending from the cell body. There are two types of extending fibres–axons and dendrites.

Dendrites look like little tree branches and receive impulses, and carry them towards the cell body and across it.

Axons are longer and carry the impulse away from the cell body to another neuron or to a muscle or a gland. They are a single fibre extending from the cell body, and can be really quite long. In some cases it maybe as long as the spinal column (the top of the neck to the sacrum (where you sit), or from the spinal cord to a foot. Some are much shorter, only connecting from one neuron in the brain to another. The axons divide at the end.

Raise your right arm. Don't worry, we're not in court. Extend your fingers. They are like dendrites picking up neurotransmitters fired across synapses. They carry an impulse towards the palm of your hand—that's the cell body. If enough dendrites convey an impulse towards the cell body, your palm, then the cell will fire an impulse down the axon—your arm. The analogy breaks down here, because at the end of the axon, there are divisions into little branches, all ending in little 'buds' or axon terminals. In the terminals are mini pockets, or 'vesicles' housing chemicals called neurotransmitters.

When an impulse reaches the end of the axon, the neurotransmitters are released, and they fire across the tiny space the synapse, to be picked up by dendrites from another neuron... and so the transmission continues. Around the body, neurons that terminate at junctions on muscle fibres cause muscles to contract. Within the brain, neurons fire to stimulate more neurons generating patterns of activity within specialised areas and between associated areas.

Some axons are coated by a fatty substance called 'myelin'. It protects the fibre and acts as an insulator a bit like the way the coloured plastic sheaths insulate electrical wires around your home. There are little gaps or 'nodes' along the myelin sheath.

The myelin sheath and these gaps or nodes are important because they speed up conduction of nerve impulses. The impulse, instead of having to travel along the length of the axon relatively slowly (I said 'relatively', actually, it's all incredibly fast), jumps from node to node, so skips most of the journey.

In Multiple Sclerosis, as we shall see later, there are patches in the CNS where myelin is disrupted, interfering with the smooth and speedy normal transmission of signals. This means the brain sends a signal to move a group of muscles, to walk for example, and it doesn't properly get through. Sometimes it might not get through at all!

There are three types of neurons. Sensory neurons carry signals from the rest of the body to the CNS. That's how the brain gets to know about pain, how your body is orientated, what you can see, hear, smell, taste, and touch. You wouldn't be aware of any of this without the signals coming in to the central control along sensory neurons. Then there are 'interneurons', or 'association fibres' that relay signals from one part of the CNS to the other, sometimes only a very tiny distance, or in the case of a large bundle of these neurons called the 'Corpus Callosum', between the two halves of the brain, left and right. This helps the different areas of your brain to communicate and co-ordinate a response to those incoming signals. And then there are 'motor' neurons. These carry signals to muscles, organs and glands so that the body is stimulated to take the appropriate action decided in the CNS in response to the sensory signals.

Nerves

The neurons we've been discussing are grouped into bundles just like the wires in a cable all over the body. Within the brain and spinal column (the CNS) the 'cables' are called tracts. In the PNS, the rest of the nervous system, they're called 'nerves'.

A nerve might contain only motor neurons, or only sensory neurons, or a mixture of both, just as a road could be a one-way street, or a motorway with traffic going in both directions. So, we can have sensory nerves, motor nerve or mixed nerves. Each neuron though, (an individual 'wire' in the 'cable') only carries signals one way—it is either a sensory or a motor neuron. It is just as on the motorway, we don't have traffic going both ways in the same lane.

Sending Signals

Between the end of an 'axon' of one nerve cell, and the ends of the branches of the tree-like 'dendrites' of the next cell, (Fig 1.1) there is a very small space called a 'synapse' (Fig 1.2). An electrical stimulus reaching the axon end causes small pockets or 'vesicles' to release a chemical called a 'neurotransmitter' into the space or synapse. Some of the chemical just floats around, some is picked up by receptors on the dendrites of the next cell, and some is taken up again by the axon that fired it.

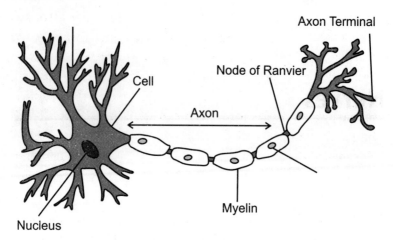

Fig. 1.1 : 'Neuron' or 'Nerve cell'

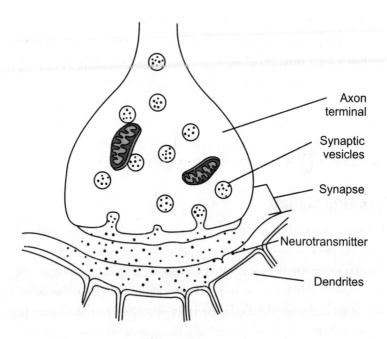

Fig. 1.2 : 'A synapse'

Some of the conditions we will be discussing are associated with a depletion of some of the chemicals or 'neurotransmitters' that ought to be firing across synapses in certain parts of the brain- that is, specialised cells that should be firing particular neurotransmitters die off. **Parkinson's disease, Huntington's disease and Alzheimer's disease** are examples of this. In Parkinson's, cells that produce a neurotransmitter called 'dopamine' are affected. Dopamine plays an important role in initiating movement, and maintaining steady control of the movement, especially in the 'substantia nigra' an area in the midbrain, part of the 'basal nuclei'.

Treatments for Alzheimer's disease have been based on the theory that depletion of cells producing another neurotransmitter, acetylcholine, is the cause of the disease. This view has proved to be controversial, as we shall see in the section on Alzheimer's disease. The relationship between neurotransmitters and Huntington's disease maybe particularly complex (Romero et al, 2008).

The Brain and the Spinal Cord

The three mothers, snugly wrapped around the brain and the spinal cord (the central nervous system or CNS) are three membranes (thin protective layers). The innermost, in contact with the brain and spinal cord is known as the Pia Mater. This means the 'tender mother'. It delicately supports and contains many tiny blood vessels, and cradling the home of our consciousness, and our very sense of being. Around that, the middle layer is the arachnoid mater. Again it is delicate, with spider-web-like fibres, giving the layer it's name (in the Greek legend the goddess Athena challenged a girl named Arachne to a weaving contest. Arachne won. Athena was angry and turned Arachne into a spider. The Latin name for spiders is arachnoids). And the outer layer is the dura mater or 'tough mother'. On the outside, the protection needs to be tough. Of course, an even tougher mother protects the brain over the dura mater—the skull. These three thin protective layers are called the meninges.

Cerebrospinal Fluid

Inside the brain are four cavities or 'ventricles'. Two, known as the lateral ventricles sit side by side pretty much in the middle of the brain divided by only a thin membrane. And the third is central beneath them, and the fourth just under that, a little towards the back. They interconnect and are filled with a special fluid called cerebrospinal fluid or CSF. The whole brain and spinal cord are bathed in this protective fluid.

The Brain

The large body of the brain is known as the cerebrum.

The 'brainstem', that leads from the top of the spinal cord and widens to become the base of the brain is divided into three parts—the medulla oblongata nearest to the spinal cord, and the pons (the word means bridge) in the middle, and the midbrain at the top.

Cerebrum

As said, it's the biggest part of the brain. It is divided into two hemispheres left and right and these are separated by a deep fissure or crevice. The cerebrum bears some resemblance to a huge walnut not that I've ever seen such a huge walnut. If you haven't looked at a walnut for quite sometime, do get one and have a look.

If you manage to crack the shell carefully, you may find the nut in two halves and intact. (I told you this book would give you the subject in a nutshell!). Skilfully extract one half. This is your model cerebrum—not perfect by any means. Hold it in front of you with the flatter surface facing down, so that you're looking at the crinkly rounded surface with the fissure running straight ahead.

The cerebrum is divided into eight lobes or sections, four in each half. Furthest from you are the frontal lobes. Some call the piece at the very front the prefrontal lobes. On top in the middle as you look down on your walnut are the parietal lobes. To the side under those lobes are the temporal lobes. And at the back you have the occipital lobes. That gives you a very rough idea where the lobes are, but of course, your model does not have the fissures that clearly mark the boundaries of each lobe. But now that you have a feel for the general location, you can check out the diagram in **Fig 1.3**.

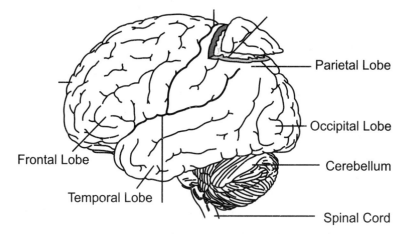

Fig. 1.3: Outer structure of the brain

The outer part of the cerebrum is called the cortex. It's surface is made up of cell bodies giving it a darkish colour – 'grey matter'. Inside the cerebrum, beneath the grey matter surface, the lobes are connected with a mass of 'white matter' tracts of white nerve fibres. Picture your walnut back in position. At the bottom of the deep fissure or crevice, the two halves are connected by a sort of bridge. In the brain, a large body of white fibres make up that bridge and carry impulses from one half of the brain to the other in both directions. In fact it is called the huge body, or in Latin, 'corpus callosum' (corpus = similar to corpse- body, and it's colossal).

Generally and simplistically speaking, the activity going on in the cerebral cortex, the outer layer of the cerebrum, with all its folds, wrinkles and fissures, give rise to what we are conscious of—thoughts, perceptions and so on. But we are not conscious of activity going on beneath the cortex controlling many body functions. I find it strange that while the cortex activity results in consciousness and awareness of so much going on all around us we are not conscious or aware of any of the activity itself. The activities going on in the cortex are to do with:

1. *Mental activity:* This includes memory, thinking, a sense of learning, intelligence and a sense of morality.

2. *Perception:* The cortex makes sense of incoming sensory information and allows us to perceive pain, temperature, sight, sound, touch, taste and smell. It's easy to imagine how frightening and unpredictable the world must be, if it is no longer possible to make sense of the information coming in, or if the sense you do make by putting patchy pieces of what you see, hear, feel and taste is inaccurate. This happens in many conditions including **stroke** and **dementia**, which we will go into later.

3. *Voluntary motor control of skeletal muscles:* There are many conditions with a motor disorder such as **dystonia** and **spasticity**, some of which are due to a problem here in the cerebral cortex. But sometimes the problem lies deeper in the cerebrum or elsewhere in the nervous system.

The Lobes

I mentioned briefly above that the cerebrum is partially divided by deep fissures into eight lobes, four in each half—the frontal, parietal, temporal and occipital lobes.

Frontal Lobe

The highest levels of thinking and intelligence occur in the frontal lobes. Changing your mind because someone points out that another approach is more reasonable, seeing things from someone else's point of view, and keeping a lid on impulses like hitting someone, or making sexual advances for example, require activity in the frontal lobe.

Just think for a minute how you might behave if because of some damage in the frontal lobe, you could no longer contain impulses, and had to say or act on every thought that crossed your mind! Some people with damage here do manage to avoid being inappropriate in public, but the sheer effort of having to actively keep a grip on social behaviour is exhausting, and sometimes once back at home and trying to relax in familiar company, it is no longer possible to contain it at all. Family caregivers suffer, but this is also terribly upsetting for the care receiver who really can't help the behaviour at all. Many conditions can lead to frontal lobe problems leaving people unable to contain these impulses or change a line of thinking or see another person's point of view. We can talk about ways of dealing with these problems later.

Also, the frontal lobes are involved in language production, working memory (aspects of memory including working memory will be considered further on), motor function (controlling body movement), sexual behaviour, problem solving, facial movement and motivation.

Mature 'adult' thinking depends on maturation of cerebral fibres in the frontal lobes and this tends to occur between late teens and mid twenties. The white matter in the frontal lobes contains more myelin than in the teen years, while the grey matter in the parietal and temporal lobes is mature by the teens. **Schizophrenia** in early adult years is associated with poorly myelinated axons linking the cells in the fore-brain.

Remember, we had discussed how the firing of electrical impulses involves chemicals called neurotransmitters being fired from the end of a neuron's axon, across a gap—a 'synapse' and picked up by those branch-like 'dendrites'? Well, there are a lot of different neurotransmitters, and we will come to them later. One important neurotransmitter is called 'dopamine'. Further on, I will say a little about how the 'thalamus' (a mass of cells deep within the brain) is involved in controlling which signals coming in from the senses are allowed along a pathway to the cortex which is the outer layer of the grey matter and the conscious part of the brain. Well, the pathways from the thalamus to the frontal cortex use dopamine, and this plays an important role in giving rise to pleasure, motivation, being able to plan and a long term memory. Problems with the regulation of dopamine pathways are known to be associated with **schizophrenia**. Thoughts are so active, it is difficult to distinguish between imagination and reality.

The frontal area is also involved in making choices about the best course of action and being aware of the likely future consequences of decisions. If you look back over these functions associated with the frontal lobes of the brain, you can see why people who have damage in that area, perhaps because of a **stroke** or frontal traumatic **head injury** often seem to behave so socially unacceptably, so impulsively, without apparent regard for the way they make others feel, or anything that might happen as a result of what they do. They tend to be unsafe because their ability to judge a risk is impaired.

The major problem for people with problems related to the frontal lobes is that the people around them tend to find it difficult to be empathetic, and get easily annoyed with them. That's because, if the rest of the brain is relatively unscathed, their IQ is probably unaffected. 'Concrete' thinking is still intact. So you may well play a game of chess with them, and have a good conversation about factual topics, and their memory can seem good. In fact, you maybe made to feel a bit foolish if you do something a bit absent minded as they may well pick you up on it. So you're possibly not going to want to cut them the slack that you might allow someone who was much more obviously confused.

It can be infuriating to find that someone apparently so intelligent is not prepared to see a situation your way and acts so seemingly selfishly. Just remember at those times, 'concrete' thinking might be all right, but it's the abstract stuff like putting themselves in someone else's shoes, that just cannot be done. (Actually, games like chess will become more difficult, as the ability to guess the other player's next move is impaired).

It's not their fault when they can't see someone else's point of view and look at it their way. They're not being awkward. But if you're annoyed by it, forgive yourself— that's natural. Hopefully, being able to have some kind of picture of what has happened to the brain to cause this behaviour, it becomes a little more possible to avoid taking it personally and to be empathetic. It should be a lot easier for us nurses, than for family caregivers. We at least go home when the shift is over! But I'm not playing down how difficult this work can be at times for all. It can also be incredibly rewarding.

The Parietal Lobes

The Parietal lobes sit above the occipital lobes and the temporal lobes behind the frontal lobes as you see in the diagram, **Fig 1.3**. Less is known about the functions of this lobe than the other three in each half (or hemisphere) of the cortex. But it does have a lot to do with integrating the information received from all the senses. In other words, making a coherent understanding of the experience of being in the surrounding world from the clues, or pieces of the jigsaw that can be seen, heard, felt, tasted, and smelt and perceived in more subtle ways. We tend to take this well orchestrated presentation of our world for granted, but try to think for a moment, how frightening the world might seem, if all this incoming information remained fragmented (or dis-integrated). This is the kind of world the people with parietal lobe damage may find themselves living in.

A particular aspect of this role in integrating sensory information is in commanding what is referred to as spatial awareness and navigation. Putting together information about the physical orientation of the body; where your arms and legs are pointing for example (without you having to look) with information about the layout of the room, the street, the stairs, whatever, making it possible to relax and trust that you can navigate around confidently.

The Temporal Lobes

Sitting under the parietal lobe, behind the frontal lobe, and in front of the occipital lobe in each hemisphere is the temporal lobe (**Fig 1.3**). In other words, they lie at the two lower sides of the brain. The brain is said here to look like a boxing glove. So it does. Forget my walnut for a minute. The part where the fingers would be protected is the frontal lobe. The parietal lobes sits above the back of the hand, with the occipital lobe over the back of the wrist, and the temporal lobe is where the thumb would be.

Functions of the temporal lobe include activity in processing what you hear, and making sense of language (both what you hear and what you plan to say) and to vision. Deeper within the temporal lobe lies the hippocampus which has a very important role in forming and maintaining memories.

In the left temporal lobe, a small specialised area known as Wernicke's area has a specific function related to speech. It seems to make sense of what needs to be said, and organises the thoughts into coherent sense, ready for processing into words to be delivered. This final stage in the process, where the words are actually formed and the mechanism to utter them put in place occurs in an adjacent area, that is actually located next door in the frontal lobe and is known as Broca's area.

So, if a **stroke** occured in Wernicke's area, the person maybe able to form words and say them clearly, but they may not make any sense. On the other hand if Wernicke's area is intact and Broca's area is affected, the person may know what he is trying to say, but can't get the words out.

In a similar way to how thoughts are made meaningful and organised coherently ready for speech, so the temporal lobe makes sense of and processes auditory information coming into the ears, so that it can be understood or interpreted.

Specialised areas around the underside of the temporal lobe are involved in visual processing, enabling objects and faces to be recognised. It is important to realise that different areas process each of these (objects and faces) and that even within these aspects of recognition there are further distinctions. Sometimes a **stroke** leaves a person able to recognise what an object is and name it, yet unable to say what it would be used for. Another person may recognise what the object is for but cannot name it. One person may recognise that a face is indeed a face, and maybe able to say whether the expression is happy, sad, angry or disgusted, yet maybe unable to recognise who the face belongs to, even if it is of a loved one. This could happen as a result of a stroke and tends to happen in **Alzheimer's disease**.

On the other hand, a stroke in a nearby area may leave those abilities intact but may leave the affected person able to say who the face belongs to, but would have no idea what sort of expression the face was wearing. This also tends to happen in **Huntington's disease**, where in particular the look of disgust has been shown to be difficult to identify.

Memory will be considered later, but for now, it is worth mentioning that there are different types of memory. Procedural memory refers to your ability to remember how to do things you have learned, perhaps for example, how to walk, run, ride a bike, play the piano, type, tie a shoelace, wash, dress, shave, clean your teeth or eat and drink without choking or spilling food. That kind of memory involves a different area of the brain, the basal nuclei which is described below. The middle area of the temporal lobe however, seems to have an important role in what is called 'episodic memory'. This is what you probably think of mostly when you consider memory—the phenomenon that you can conjure up an experience like a film clip, running through some past episode in your life.

The temporal lobes are also important in the conversion of short term memories to long term, and in memories of where things are in relation to one another, including spatial memory.

Occipital Lobe

Most people seem to know that a bang on the back of the head over where the occipital lobe is can make you see 'stars'. This lobe processes the information coming into the brain from the optic nerve which carries impulses from the retina at the back of each eye. It makes the scene look complete and coherent, even though the eyes do not look steadily at anything, they scan very quickly back and forth and if you were to perceive what actually comes in the rawest form, it would give you a very chaotic impression of a crazy world. Test this for yourself. Look quickly at the second hand on a clock that moves every second. Look away. Repeat this several times. Every now and then, you will find that the 'second' seems to last longer. That's because though you were sure you were looking at it, you weren't. You missed the move while scanning, and had to wait to catch the next movement.

This lobe also seems to have some role in the processing of hearing. While I've tried to offer an overview of what these parts of the brain are involved in, the truth is much more complex—way beyond mere mortals like me to understand. But I do believe, as I indicated at the outset, that while such an overview might amuse an expert on brains and behaviour, for us caregivers and nurses, I feel it's a good enough level of understanding to work with. I do hope you'll find that to be the case.

The Deeper Structures of the Brain

Deep within each of the two cerebral hemispheres are three areas of masses of cell bodies, more of that darker, 'grey matter'. These three areas are identified in **Figs 1.4** and **1.5**. They are the basal nuclei, the thalamus and the hypothalamus.

The **basal nuclei** have a lot to do with coordinating smooth movements and problems here can result in jerky, uncontrolled involuntary limb and body movements, as in **Huntington's disease**, or a tremor and difficulty initiating movement as in **Parkinson's disease**. We will explore the problems in more depth further on. The basal nuclei also have connections to other parts of the brain including the cerebral cortex. So problems here can create problems elsewhere also.

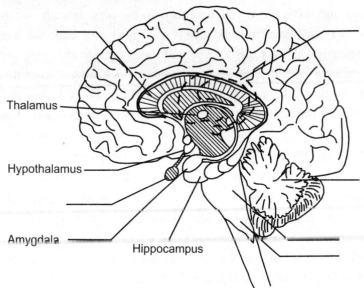

Thalamus

Hypothalamus

Amygdala

Hippocampus

Fig. 1.4 : Sagittal section of the brain

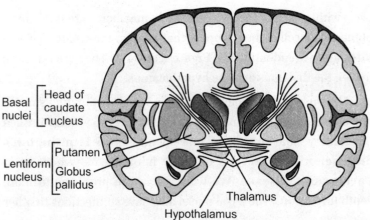

Basal nuclei { Head of caudate nucleus

Lentiform nucleus { Putamen · Globus pallidus

Thalamus

Hypothalamus

Fig. 1.5 : Coronal section of the brain

The **thalamus** acts as a sort of gate control. It is in two halves, thinly joined in the middle of the two halves of the cerebrum. All the sensory information coming from everywhere around the body, except the sense of smell, comes via this mass of junctions (synapses, as we discussed previously). It sifts all this incoming information and decides what should be fed up to the cortex, where we will become conscious of it, and what should not.

Have you ever been to a cocktail party where a large room full of people are chatting? You can't hear what any of them are saying in the background as someone starts chatting to you. Then across the room, someone mentions your name quietly, and you immediately home in on it?

Your thalamus picked up all the signals. You were hearing all the background chatter in detail, but not consciously. Then the decision was made that someone said something you may need to be aware of. That's why you might not wake if a family member in your house flushes the toilet at night, even though it maybe loud, but you'd quickly be alerted to a quiet footstep out in your garden. The familiar noise is no cause for concern, but you may need to know about the possible intruder. Hopefully, it's just the neighbour's cat!

The thalamus also plays a role in regulating sleep more generally, and a stroke affecting this part of the brain could cause a permanent coma.

The **hypothalamus**, just beneath the thalamus (hypo means below, beneath or low) is an area that maintains what is called the body's 'homeostasis'; that is, keeping aspects such as body temperature, blood pressure, the amount of fluid in the body, and of 'electrolytes' such as sodium and potassium within normal ranges. Health and life depend on those being kept in balance. It wouldn't take you long to consider that list of functions and the consequences in case of any damage to the hypothalamus.

So far, in considering the brain, we have discussed only the cerebrum, the very large part shaped something like a walnut. I know, it's a crude description, and there are many more parts than I have mentioned and they all work in rather more complex ways than I've suggested. But as I pointed out in the introduction, you and I aren't trying to become neurologists or neurosurgeons. We're simply trying to care for people with trouble in the central nervous system, and it just helps to have a not-too detailed map of where these problems occur from, and why in general terms, we are seeing the kind of behaviour or other problems we need to help people affected by degenerative brain disorders to compensate for.

Then we delved deeper into the brain and considered the functions of the masses of 'grey matter' within the cerebrum, the basal nuclei, the thalamus and the hypothalamus. Now let's venture further down leaving the cerebrum to the brain stem.

The Brain Stem

This section, as you might have guessed is the extension at the base of the brain, continuous with the spinal cord. It is divided into three parts.

The 'medulla oblongata', often just called the medulla, is nearest to the cerebrum. The medulla houses the respiratory centre-controlling breathing, and also reflexes such as coughing and vomiting. The vaso-motor centre is located here controlling the blood pressure, by constricting or dilating (opening / narrowing) arteries as is cardiac (heart) control.

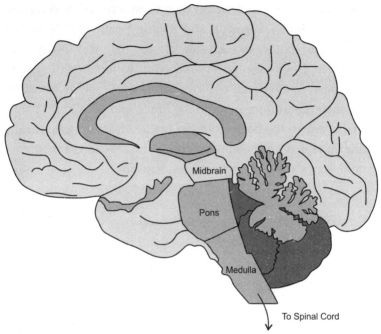

Fig. 1.6 : Brain stem

Above the medulla, is the midbrain. It serves as a pathway to the cerebral left and right hemispheres. Reflexes to auditory and visual signals arise here.

And between the medulla and the midbrain is the pons (meaning 'bridge'). It's a kind of relay station, assisting in conveying signals from the medulla to the higher centres including the cortex.

An injury to or a stroke within the brain stem would be devastating.

The Spinal Cord

Extending like a tail from the base of the brain, the spinal cord is around 45 cm long and as thick as your finger. It is protected within the vertebrae. The small round bones make up the spine. It is divided into 31 segments and at each, a pair of mixed nerves (sensory and motor) on each side left and right exit towards the outer body. The outer edges of the cord are white tracts (the axons of neurons) of motor and sensory nerves conveying information from the body and sense up to the brain, and sending response signals back to the body from the brain. An inner, grey area is made up of nerve cell bodies. Within a cross section of the spinal cord this grey matter is shaped like a butterfly.

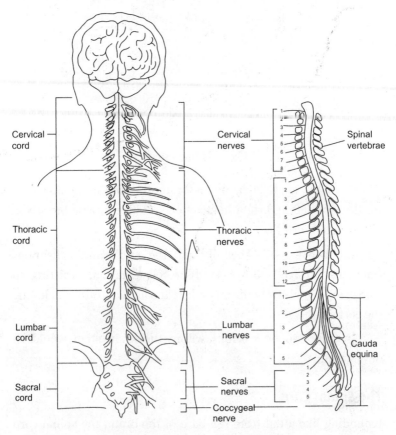

Fig. 1.7 : Spinal cord and spinal nerves

Sensory information coming from say a heat or pain centre in the hand can loop within the spinal cord, to stimulate a motor nerve which will carry an impulse to appropriate muscle causing contraction so that the hand moves away quickly. Meanwhile, the pain or heat sensory information will be carried up to the brain where it is perceived. But already the evasive action has been taken. You took your hand off the hotplate before you felt the heat.

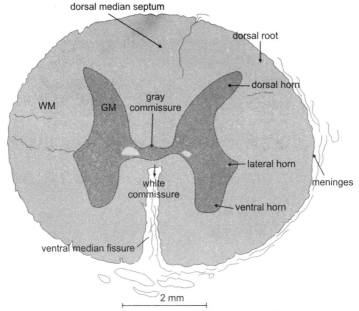

Fig. 1.8 : Cross section of the spinal cord

There you are! In a nutshell—that's the central nervous system.

Thank you for bearing with the anatomy and physiology section. It may have seemed a bit of a chore, although I don't feel you need to remember it all by any means. Don't worry at all if you can't remember any. I think you'll find this background information helpful as we discuss the neurological disorders and how they affect people in the following sections.

I should say that these are brief outlines, just to give us an idea, so that we can then go on to discuss generally, caring for people with any of these neurological conditions, knowing that most of the challenges we face are shared across the diagnoses, while some things are fairly specific to particular disorders.

PART B
DIAGNOSES

Parkinson's Disease

Parkinson's disease (PD) is a complex, fluctuating condition. Often people around someone with PD don't understand this important point, and therefore can find it difficult to appreciate why things that are easy to do on one occasion can be almost impossible at another time. Each person with PD is affected differently and individually. The condition will progress at different rates in different people. Each will have a different medication regimen that will need to be adhered to at times specific to the individual. This is so important, and is why the concept of a 'drug round' (that is, administering prescribed drugs to patients starting at one end of the ward, and working systematically to the far end, rather than individually giving his or her medicine at the right time for that person) is a bad idea with regard to people with PD. Many people involved in nursing or caring for people with PD are not fully aware of this.

Parkinson's disease can be difficult to identify in its early stages, because it is closely related to other diagnoses characterised by similar signs. It is one of a group of neurological conditions known as 'movement disorders'. The four major signs of PD are tremor, slow movement, rigidity and postural instability.

Having some symptoms similar to those seen in PD does not by any means then, indicate that it is PD. 'Parkinsonism' can result as a side effect of some medications, for example, anti psychotic medications and the symptoms may subside if medication is discontinued or changed with the help of the prescribing physician. So called 'recreational' drugs can induce parkinsonism in some people, and it can also result from a stroke. Some other conditions associated with very similar symptoms are mentioned a little further on.

But it can also be seen as occurring, I take the view, as a normal sign of aging. I noticed on my 45th birthday, when my dad kindly sent me a cheque to choose a book with, that his signature had become smaller and rather shaky. He was 79 and when I visited him later in the year, I observed that, sure enough, his right hand had developed a slight resting tremor, and that it had got better, but was still there, when he carried out fine motor tasks such as writing. I'm sure this would have developed slowly, but I wouldn't call it any kind of disease; he was getting older and cells in a variety of places were no doubt degenerating. He died a year later of an unrelated condition.

In contrast my dear aunt did have PD. Otherwise, healthy in her mid 60's, her left handed tremor became a nuisance, which was not just noticeable in handwriting. Both the arms and gradually all her limbs were affected quite severely. The stiffness all through her body and the slowed movement made it hard to carry out her usual daily chores. She was such a busy, outgoing fun loving aunt that it was hard to accept these increasing limitations. She had been a speedy typist, and that became out of the question. Everything wore her out—the sheer effort of washing, dressing, eating, and getting to the shops. Eventually she did everything with her devoted husband's help.

One night, while heading for the toilet, she fell and sustained a nasty injury that resulted in hospitalisation. She had surgery for deep brain stimulation, on one side of her head. The neurosurgeon was very pleased with the result. According to his assessment, the tremor and rigidity on one side of her body was much improved. He suggested a second operation of the other side. My aunt was not so impressed with the result. She felt more disabled than ever, and would not entertain any more surgery. This was about ten years ago. Since then interest among professionals in 'patient reported outcomes and patient perceived quality of life' as measures of the effectiveness of interventions has increased, and become as important as clinical, objective measures (Pablo et al 2008). We now appreciate more that what maybe extremely helpful to one person, may not suit another, and patients are central to decisions about their care and treatment. Certainly for many people with PD, deep brain stimulation has been a fabulous intervention.

Parkinson's affects people very individually. Some people are unaffected as my dad with his barely noticeable tremor, or as badly impacted and debilitated as my dear aunt.

The tremor in PD generally begins on one side, typically seen in one hand. Movement of the finger and thumb rhythmically back and forth is descriptively known as 'pill-rolling'. This 'unilateral' presentation can help to distinguish PD from anxiety, or effects of some medications in which a similar tremor tends to appear on both sides. For most people with PD (70% according to Factor and Weiner, 2002) the tremor is the first noticed indication of the condition and classically occurs at rest. The tremor in PD increases over time and progresses from the hand up to the arm. Typically it spreads to the opposite arm or to the leg on the same side. Eventually, all limbs, the jaw and face are involved. However, the pace of the progression is very individual, with some people finding that the tremor remains in one hand for years, and others affected bilaterally fairly rapidly.

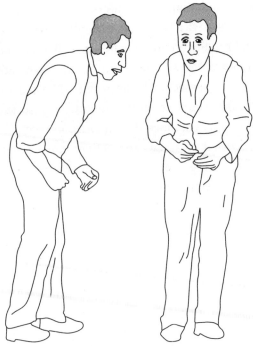

Fig. 2.1 : Parkinson's disease

The stiffness, or rigidity affects all limbs and the torso. It is a resistance to movement, and is often seen in one arm and the neck in early stages of PD, progressing to both sides. It can be what is called 'lead pipe' rigidity, where the resistance to passive movement is even, or 'cogwheel' rigidity- intermittent; as though on a ratchet. Both tremor and rigidity may fluctuate in severity during any day and are often exacerbated by stress. So, trying to hurry the person along tends to be counterproductive, and exercising patience really pays off.

The term often used to describe the slowness in movement is 'bradykinesia'—'brady' meaning slow and 'kinetics' is to do with body movement. While the tremor maybe the most noticeable feature of PD, bradykinesia is the most disabling symptom. It is also the most frustrating aspect.

Postural instability, or impaired balance and coordination is another highly disabling feature of PD.

Together, these symptoms increasingly make activities such as walking and talking, dressing, washing, managing to get to the toilet on time and eating difficult, as the disease progresses.

Added to these problems, many people with PD suffer from depression and other emotional disturbance. The so called 'non-motor' symptoms are sometimes referred to as 'the other side of Parkinson's' and frequently people complain that these aspects can be more disturbing than the motor disorder itself. Skin problems may occur; sleep can be disrupted and there can be specific problems with urination and constipation, swallowing, chewing and speaking.

Typically, the voice becomes a 'monotone'—flat and without intonation. Facial muscles have impaired tone and so there is limited expression. This can make communication very difficult and frustrating, and it well help caregivers to know that the lack

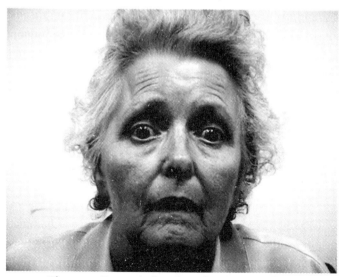

Fig. 2.2 : Expressionless face of Parkinson's disease

of body language such as a smile doesn't mean a lack of interest or humour or gratitude. Communication difficulties can often lead to social isolation.

The diagnosis is based on medical history and neurological examination. The consultant may give advice for brain scans or laboratory tests to rule out other conditions but there are no laboratory tests to diagnose PD. Conditions associated with similar movement disorder problems to those seen in PD include:

Multiple system atrophy (MSA)—A rare degenerative neurological condition presenting with low blood pressure as well as 'parkinsonism' (Parkinson's type symptoms), occurring mostly over the age of 55.

Progressive Supranuclear Palsy (PSP) (or Steele Richardson— Olszewski syndrome, after the doctors who identified the disease) is a comparatively rapidly progressing disease with personality change often occurring early, and with eye movement problems, often leading to falls.

Dementia with Lewy bodies (DLB)—This condition is discussed later, but briefly, Lewy Bodies are round masses developing in cell bodies in the brain and displace other important cell components. Many people with PD are cognitively unaffected... they don't get any noticeable signs of dementia. But there is a clear association between DLB and PD that is, a significant number of people with PD develop DLB.

The Causes of PD

Causes of Parkinson's disease are complex. There isn't a single route cause as there is with the next condition we will consider-Huntington's disease, which is caused by a fault in a single gene. (Actually even that maybe a little more complex). But PD tends to be put down to multi-factorial causes.

There does seem to be a genetic factor. In some families where PD is prevalent, there is a shared genetic mutation. But this is a small number of families and most people with PD don't have the identified mutation. There is a general consensus though that young-onset PD is genetically inherited. Some external environmental factors have been implicated in the cause of PD such as exposure to carbon monoxide and some pesticides.

You may have heard people talk about 'free radicals' causing diseases in all sorts of contexts. This is thought to be a factor in PD. As you may know, a molecule, the basic structure of the material that we (and the world around us) are made of, consist of atoms. The number of positively charged particles (protons) in the atom's nucleus determines how many negatively charged particles (electrons) orbit around the atom. If the outer 'shell' has a full complement of electrons orbiting, it doesn't interact with other atoms, but when the numbers of protons and electrons is unbalanced, atoms do interact to restore stability by sharing electrons, or by one electron being picked up by the other atom. Sometimes this process can leave a molecule in an unbalanced situation, and this then becomes a 'free radical'. By interacting with other molecules and destabilising their balance between positive and negative charge, further free radicals are created.

So, this process also seems to be an important factor that breaks down cells that should produce and utilise dopamine, in the striata nigra, an area in the midbrain, and part of the basal nuclei. (These areas, with a crucial role in smooth movement and coordination were discussed earlier, and depletion of these dopamine-producing cells is the underlying problem in Parkinson's disease).

A history of a head injury and repeated knocks to the head as experienced by many boxers, even if they are as good at dodging punches as Muhamed Ali was, are said to be causal also.

For whatever reason the dopamine producing cells are depleted, and when about only 80% are left intact, signs of PD start to become noticeable (so probably the disease process began years before this) and as they continue to be destroyed, symptoms will progress.

It maybe worth looking back at the section on 'sending signals' if you feel a bit rusty about 'synapses', 'neurotransmitters' and 'dopamine'.

Treatment for Parkinson's Disease

As is generally the case with the degenerative neurological conditions discussed in this book, there is no 'cure' for Parkinson's disease, but some treatments are effective. Particularly in PD, some medications do have a dramatic positive effect. Having said it, the response is rather individual. Ask anyone who has type 1 diabetes what the treatment is, and they'll say 'insulin', or try someone with asthma, and the first answer is nearly always their ventolin inhaler. That's because these work predictably and very effectively in pretty much all cases.

Try asking ten people with back pain or depression the most effective treatment and you'll possibly get 10 different answers. When there are a lot of treatments for a condition, you can pretty much bet that none of them answer the problems for everyone. But that isn't to say that finding the right way forward for an individual can't improve life dramatically—it can. There are a lot of approaches to treating the symptoms of PD. Some are medical (that is, drugs), some are surgical (that is, involve an operation) and some are less physically invasive.

Drugs

The aims of drug therapies for PD are to increase the amount of dopamine getting to the brain, to optimise the effect of the dopamine that is in the brain and to interfere with other neurotransmitters and enzymes that have an effect on the way dopamine can work in the brain.

In the early stages of PD, physicians tend to be very cautious about introducing medication, and advise reducing the severity and the impact of the symptoms by conservative means including maintaining a healthy diet and lifestyle, exercising and relaxing.

For an excellent, comprehensive and easy to understand explanation of the drugs used to treat Parkinson's disease, read the booklet entitled 'Drug treatment of Parkinson's disease, for people living with Parkinson's', available from the Parkinson's Disease Society (2008), and see the references which are downloadable. There is no point in attempting to reproduce such a helpful resource here, and so only a very brief outline of what some of the main drugs do is provided with the strong recommendation to access the booklet. This is only a very brief overview and it must be noted that decisions about medication should be informed by discussion with the physician, and the manufacturer's instructions must be followed.

Levodopa began greatly improving the lives of many people with PD in the 1960s. Madopar (co-beneldopa) and sinemet (co-careldopa) are the most common preparations, both containing an extra substance to prevent levodopa being changed to dopamine before reaching the brain, because dopamine cannot cross the blood-brain barrier that is, it would not access the brain if it were transformed too early.

Madopar and Sinemet are started in a low dose, and gradually titrated upwards until both patient and doctor are agreed that there is a satisfactory response. Dispersible Madopar (in water) is absorbed quickly, and is helpful to some patients who do not have a good result from slower release preparations, and to some who have problems with swallowing as a result of their PD. The letters 'CR' following the drug name (for example, sinemet CR) indicate a 'controlled release' preparation. This prolongs the time it takes for the drug to be absorbed, and suits some people with PD who have problems related to the good effect of the drug wearing off prior to the following dose. Taken at night for example, for some, a CR preparation can enhance comfort and sleep until morning, and make movement easier for example, if the person needs to get up in the night for the toilet.

While many people with PD tolerate Madopar and Sinemet very well, and experience a great reduction in debilitating symptoms, for a minority side effects can include sickness, confusion, hallucinations and serious mood swings.

Over the years, the benefits of Levodopa can begin to wear off, with the effects of one dose failing to last sufficiently until the next. There can be sudden changes between being able to mobilise (the 'on' phase) and unable to move (the 'off' phase). There can also be unwanted, involuntary jerky movements as the levels of dopamine activating movement fluctuate within the brain.

For some people with PD, adversely affected by these effects, 'dopamine agonists' provide a suitable answer. These are drugs that imitate the action of dopamine by stimulating cells in the same way that dopamine does. They are sometimes used alone for people with newly diagnosed PD. They are not generally as effective as levodopa, but carry less tendency towards side effects. For people who have used sinemet or madopar and have begun to experience side effects, a dopamine agonist can be used with their other medication as an adjunct.

These medications include Ropinirole hydrochloride; Pergolide mesilate and Bromocriptine mesylate. They must be introduced gradually as there can be unwanted effects such as nausea and vomiting, drowsiness and dizziness, confusion and hallucinations and movement problems that already exist can be exacerbated in some cases. As indicated at the beginning of this section, the choice of drugs is individual and based on very careful trial and error necessitating low doses initially.

Another dopamine agonist is apomorphine, which while most of the agonists are tablets or capsules to be taken through the mouth, can be given as an injection (some carry an apomorphine 'pen' to inject as a top up between regular medication) or as a steady infusion under the skin. Apomorphine can bring stability to people with rapid fluctuations in ability and whose 'off' periods (spells of immobility) are prolonged. It is taken with domperidone at least initially, as this drug acts to prevent sickness which can occur with apomorphine, particularly when starting to use.

Another type of drug works to block an enzyme that breaks down levodopa. These are called COMT inhibitors, for example, Entacapone (Comtess). It is taken with levodopa to maximise the effect. Another preparation, Tolcopone (Tasmar) contains levodopa, carbodopa and entacapone. Only experienced specialists prescribe this and patients need regular checks to ensure the medication is not affecting liver function. The risk of side effects is that because of the prolonged life of levodopa, its action maybe excessive, causing involuntary movement, and nausea and vomiting.

MAO-B inhibitors (for example, selegiline; rasagiline) breaks down another enzyme (monoamine oxidase), that acts to destroy dopamine in the brain. It maybe used on its own in the early stages of PD, but when taken with sinemet or madopar, it can lead to an excessive dopamine reaction including involuntary movement and resulting falls, and sometimes hallucinations, headaches and depression. It should not be taken alongside antidepressant medication such as fluoxitine. Once again, a drug option that works well with only some patients.

Amantadine is a 'glutamate inhibitor' and prolongs the effect of dopamine as well as aiding its release from cells. It has relatively few side effects but only seems to be effective in a small minority of patients. For those few though it can be a useful option.

There are other medical approaches, but these are the most common. It is worth repeating here the value of downloading the PDS booklet as referred to above, for a fuller, very helpful discussion of all the relevant medications, with their advantages and potential disadvantages and advice about taking them and contraindications.

The points to appreciate are that as the condition progresses, medication will need to be increased. It is important therefore to regularly monitor changes and be prepared to adjust the 'care package' or 'programme' accordingly. Ask for a medication review when any changes are noticed or when there is an event such as a fall. It has been said above, but it is very important to be aware that medication should be given at set time when required, and not when convenient for the caregiver. At home that's not usually a problem, but I hate to say, it's when the person with PD is admitted to a hospital or a nursing home that these problems can crop up if staff members are not aware of the importance. Time spent establishing a friendly rapport with the team and checking they all understand is worthwhile. Of course they want to get it right once they know it can't be just part of 'the 8 o'clock round'.

Debbie Chinman, who works for the Parkinson's Disease Society, frequently talks to care staff at nursing homes, uses a very helpful analogy, which she apparently got from a friend who considers that his body is like a car. The parts of a car maybe working perfectly. But when there's no diesel (not enough dopamine) he has to 'fill up the tank' (take his medication). This gets him going again. When drivers know that the car is going low on fuel, it's not a good idea to wait till the car stops altogether. You need to go to the garage and top up at once. Similarly, drugs in PD are timed so that the next dose saves everything from starting to slow down, and then causing problems getting back to normal functioning again. If the next dose is left too long, the person is likely to start to stiffen and experience rigidity. It will be a bad, frustrating day, and unnecessarily so.

Freezing

'Freezing' is a fairly common phenomenon in Parkinson's disease. The person suddenly stops when walking or wants to start walking and just can't move off the spot. It feels like the feet are 'frozen', or stuck solid to the ground. Other activities can be frozen too- such as speaking, trying to move from a seat or reach for something.

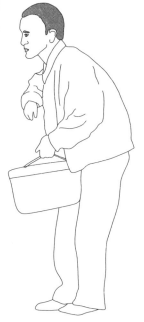

When it occurs in walking, the pace often becomes a shuffle of increasingly short steps (called 'festination') prior to the sudden stop. Freezing tends to occur with a change in the environment such as a doorway, the edge of a carpet, a change of pattern in the flooring, or going through an archway in the garden. The same person may often walk past all these types of potential triggers without problem.

The cause isn't really understood, but it can happen more frequently in

Fig. 2.3 : Freezing phenomena of Parkinson's disease

people who have been treated a long time with levodopa. These people can experience 'off' and 'on' periods. During an 'on' period, the levodopa works well and mobility is good, but during an 'off' period movement is more problematic; the drug just doesn't seem to be working! Freezing is more common in 'off' periods. When that is the case, working with the doctor to change drug timings carefully may help. But when freezing tends to occur regardless of 'off' or 'on' periods, changing medication doesn't tend to help.

If this is a problem, seek help from a physiotherapist and an occupational therapist who can help with physical techniques or consider changes to the environment or footwear that maybe helpful.

Some people find that when 'frozen', shifting weight from the left leg to the right and back, side to side, gets the movement going again, rather than trying to go forward initially. It might be helpful for some to keep stamping when getting to a doorway, to keep some momentum going while waiting to get through. Telling yourself- '1,2,3,go' can help to get a foot going when you've decided which foot to move first. Some effectively use a 'mini metronome', a clicking device attached to the hip that helps to keep stepping in time, keeping a momentum going.

The Parkinson's Disease Society website has some very useful and more detailed information on dealing with freezing, at: http://www.parkinsons.org.uk/pdf/FS63_0308_web.pdf

In particular, they demonstrate a method of strategically placing coloured strips on the floor. This is well worth a look if you have experienced the problem.

Complementary Therapies

Many people with PD and their carers find great relief from any of a variety of complementary therapies, not as an alternative, but as an adjunct to orthodox medication. Acupuncture, aromatherapy, reiki and reflexology are examples of therapies that some feel give a tangible benefit to relieving specific symptoms and are at least relaxing. 'Conductive Education' can be helpful in movement disorders such as PD, and can target specific problems as well as prevent difficulties more generally. Given that tremor, bradykinesia and rigidity can become increasingly debilitating when stressed; therapies that induce a relaxed mind and body have obvious advantages. Generally, these are felt to be free of any unwanted effects, although care should be taken before using herbal remedies. The GP should be consulted.

Surgical Intervention

Surgery can be a suitable option for some patients depending on their symptoms. Deep brain stimulation (DBS) involves implanting electrodes into the brain and these are connected to a small device called a pulse generator. This can be programmed externally. For some people this has the effect of limiting symptoms without using the medication and therefore eliminating the risk of their side effects.

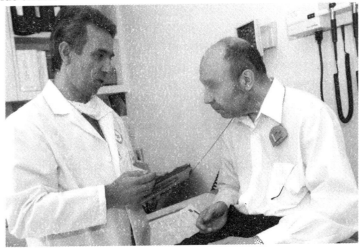

Fig. 2.4 : Deep brain stimulation

An alternative surgical procedure is more permanent and involves damaging some of the area selectively where the affected dopamine-producing neurons are. A thalamotomy involves destroying cells in the thalamus and a pallidotomy centres on the globus pallidus, part of the basal nuclei discussed in an earlier section. Research concerned with implanting stem cells to repair the damaged area, and also the infusion of chemicals into the basal nuclei is ongoing. Gene therapy is another area of research being pioneered in which new genes are inserted into cells to stimulate repair. It is too early to give predictions about the effectiveness of these approaches.

James Parkinson

It is important to mention the man who wrote the famous essay 'The Shaking Palsy' later inspiring the disease to be known by his name. He was a fascinating man with a City of London license to practice as a surgeon, and a long repertoire of publications on a variety of medical subjects including the effects of lightning, mental illness 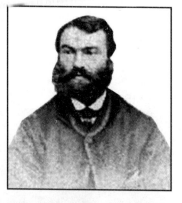 and reform and the education of medical students. He was an active social reformer and even became embroiled in a court case as a defence witness regarding accusations of a plot to kill King George III. James Parkinson lived from 1755-1824, and his write-up on the PDS website (I know I keep plugging it, but you must visit) is worth browsing.

How else can I help?

1. Staying optimistic can help. Your reaction to the person you care for having Parkinson's disease is likely to influence his or her view of it.

2. Work out with the person you care for, what he or she can do, and what is difficult because of PD. Then work out what changes might make it possible to do some of the things he or she wants to do and finds difficult.

3. A good way to help think up ideas is to break down the barriers to doing things into categories: physical barriers, psychological (or emotional) barriers, social barriers, environmental barriers, and financial barriers.

For example, Fred tells his wife, Millie, 'I miss doing the garden, I can't do it because of my Parkinson's disease.' That's a vague problem and a vague reason. We're not clear from that exactly what it is that Fred can't do; what he wants to do; or what is that which is stopping him from doing it .

Breaking the problem down Fred and Millie establish that Fred doesn't mind not mowing the lawn, or trimming the hedge, but they do need it to be done. It does annoy Fred that these are looking untidy. What he particularly misses doing is planting and digging up the vegetables and tending the flowers.

They get a pen and paper and make the category headings, ready to list the barriers to doing the gardening tasks:

Physical Barriers

Fred's unsteady gait and hand and arm tremor makes using a lawn mower or a hedge trimmer unsafe. Anyway he is fatigued by physical exertion and couldn't handle these or a pair of shears for more than a few minutes. Heavy digging is too much, but Fred feels he could dig a small patch if the ground were a little softer. He does have the strength to pull up weeds, and plant flowers and vegetables except that it can be difficult to keep bending to the ground and standing up again.

Physical Adapting

Millie points out that Fred's medications give him a few hours in the day when he's at his best. He can move more easily and suggests that's the time to be in the garden, just doing those things he can do. The important thing is to make sure the medications are taken exactly at the time prescribed, because it has taken a while to get them to give Fred this 'window of opportunity' each day. Timing is crucial they agree.

Psychological or Emotional Barriers

Fred admits that he feels defeated just thinking about doing the garden. It emphasises how little he can do compared to what he used to do, and he finds it easier just to avoid going out there.

Psychological Adapting

They discuss coming to terms with the reality that Fred can't do all that he used to. They agree that staying focussed on what Fred can't do isn't making either of them feel any better, whereas focussing on what he can do is more helpful. They agree that he used to be so busy, that although he could cut the hedge and the lawn, he never had much time to relax out there and enjoy the garden. One good consequence is that there is time now. They agree, it won't be easy to look at the positive side all the time, and when Fred, or Millie feel fed up about how things are, they should feel free to say so, and avoid bottling it up.

Social Barriers

Fred tells Millie that when he's out in the garden, he is aware of the neighbours over the fence, and is embarrassed to let them see him pottering about at a slow pace. It puts him off going out there.

Social Adapting

They decide to go and face this problem head on. They knock next door and over a cup of tea, tell the neighbours about it. The neighbours are very empathetic and understanding. Afterwards, Fred feels less self conscious about seeing them out there.

Environmental Barriers

Millie points out that they've looked at the problem of Fred finding it hard to bend down to weed and plant as a physical one, in his condition. After forcing herself to think about what about whether the environment could be the barrier, she says...'it's not that you can't reach down Fred, it's simply that the garden is too low!'

Environmental Adapting

Fred seemed perplexed, but Millie explained that if the beds with the flowers and the vegetables were raised up to his waist height, he could easily reach them.

Financial Barriers

Fred points out that raising the beds, and getting the lawn and hedge cut will cost money that is in short supply.

Financial Adapting

Millie doesn't deny it's a problem. But she says that having done this exercise, they're now clear about what will help, and if they can access any money, they know more precisely what it is needed for. They agree that they should seek advice from a social worker. Maybe there are benefits that they have not yet applied for, and are entitled to. They will contact the Parkinson's Disease Society, who might have ideas about where to try for financial help.

With that, Fred and Millie's neighbour knocks and says, 'I've been thinking, since you called in... would you feel offended if I offered to cut your hedge and mow the lawn whenever I do mine? It wouldn't be much extra, I enjoy it as it gets me out of the house. And I promise not to interfere with the vegetable and flower beds.' Fred and Millie are grateful, and agree that this answers some of the financial problem as well as improving the social aspects.

That is just an example of how problems can be clarified and tackled more systematically. In more advanced PD, problems could be around different issues. Perhaps how to stay more independent with regard to washing, dressing or shaving for example, or managing to eat a meal. Breaking any of these problems down into those same categories, barriers and ways of adapting, can help family members and nursing home staff work with the person with PD, to come up with innovative solutions. That way, medication isn't turned to as the only answer. It is part of a 'holistic' approach. 'Holistic' means taking account of the whole person, not just focussing on a physical diagnosis and treatment.

• It maybe helpful to consider joining self-help groups... not everyone's cup of tea, but many find them a life-line. Being a member of the Parkinson's Disease Society is worthwhile, and will help you keep up to date with developments and get good ideas from others. Some find that being active members opens up a new social horizon, but others prefer a very low key involvement. It's very individual and you should take the approach that suits you both best.

- It is worth contacting the Parkinson's Disease Society for a diary that they produce and the one for the carers. It can be very helpful in keeping a good, accurate and precise record of times of medications and of their effects and the disease fluctuations. This can be a very useful resource to have with you at a review with the consultant, or with the Parkinson's disease specialist nurse.

Huntington's Disease

I first encountered Huntington's disease when I worked at a nursing home for young people with neurological disorders in Scotland, run by the Sue Ryder Foundation, as 'Sue Ryder Care' was then known. Eighteen of our thirty six residents had HD. It is a devastating condition striking cruelly at individuals, and those around them, often quite reasonably causing complete breakdowns in relationships.

The symptoms of HD usually begin to manifest in midlife, perhaps between the ages of 35 and 55. There are exceptions, where onset occurs at much younger and older ages. Often, the first obvious sign is the movement disorder (chorea). This may begin with involuntary fidgety movements of the fingers, hands and feet. Sometimes these don't seem to be noticed by the individual or by close relatives. These movements are different to what is normally regarded as fidgeting but as Oliver Quarrell (2008) explains so graphically in his excellent book (see reference listed at the end of this book), the difference is hard to describe, but is easily recognised by people used to seeing it. With time the uncontrolled movements will increase, and will involve the limbs, trunk and neck. The writhing, twisting movement is known as chorea, because of its dance-like quality (chorea, from the Greek word for dance).

Other effects of HD may present simultaneously, or even earlier, but as they begin insidiously, they may not be acknowledged or even noticed till later. These include problems with cognition (thinking, calculating, memory, perception and so on), and psychiatric problems such as depression and sometimes delusions, and hallucinations. Mood swings can occur and there can be outbursts of unexplained anger. However, as we shall see later and this is true of its occurrence in relation to other neurological conditions also, sometimes these angry outbursts can be explained.

Because the cognitive problems result from the progressive loss of neurons in the brain, that is, the disease is degenerative, the term 'dementia' is sometimes used. This is not incorrect, but the loss of brain function is different to other forms of dementia such as that seen in Alzheimer's disease (AD), which is discussed in the following section. Many aspects of intelligence remain intact in HD. It is often possible to have a good intellectually stimulating conversation with someone with advanced HD. Both short and long term memory often seem remarkably sharp, and the person with HD will recognise the face of family, friends, nurses and care staff, often until the very last days.

By contrast, people with AD tend to gradually lose all cognitive ability, although despite often being unable to recognise a close family member or friend, these individuals can usually easily distinguish between a happy, sad, angry or disgusted facial expression. Research indicates that people with HD tend to have trouble recognising negative facial expressions, such as fear and disgust (Milders et al, 2003; Hennenlotter et al, 2004). This may help to explain why we don't always get the response we might expect when we show our feelings.

Despite the ability to hold his or her own in conversation (although with time, breathing and speech are affected by lost muscle control, often making communicating difficult), problems arise with flexible thinking, making plans and coping with changes in the thread of the conversation. With the progression of the disease, other problems include difficulty in inhibiting impulses. If you have ever felt angry with someone who pushed in front of you in a queue, you may have experienced an impulse to shove him or her out of the way, or worse. I'm sure it was only a fleeting thought that you didn't seriously consider acting on. The frontal part of the outer layer of your brain (frontal cortex) was involved in taking control of this impulse. In HD, the activity of this part of the brain becomes seriously affected, and it becomes increasingly difficult to inhibit such an impulse.

Equally difficult, becomes the ability to see things from another person's point of view. This also involves the frontal lobe, and is part of the higher level of thinking that we tend to regard as attributable to well-socialised human beings.

Next time you feel annoyed by seemingly impatient or selfish behaviour of a person with HD, take some time to consider what kind of person you might be, without the ability to contain the many impulses you experience each day, or to see the situation from another person's perspective. Thank goodness I have never acted upon some of my secret inner thoughts! It maybe hard to admit it, but if you're honest, you maybe able to recognise a little of yourself behind the actions you see. This mental exercise can help with accepting, and tolerating the behaviour of your client or relative (as the case maybe).

The basal ganglia, areas deep inside the brain as we have seen earlier in this book, are involved in controlling and co-ordinating movement.

This part of the brain loses so many nerve cells in HD that eventually two areas, the putamen and caudate nucleus are missing on direct examination of the brain tissue. Pathways from the basal nuclei (itself responsible for well learned motor programmes) to the frontal cortex (responsible for decisions, judgement), the cerebellum (co-ordination and balance) and motor cortex (voluntary movement) are disrupted.

One other important issue concerning people with HD is that of genetic inheritance. It has been established, above, that the symptoms of HD tend to manifest in midlife. The condition is due to a faulty gene. The inheritance pattern is dominant and the gene is 'fully penetrant'. This means that almost all carriers of the genetic fault will develop symptoms in a normal life span.

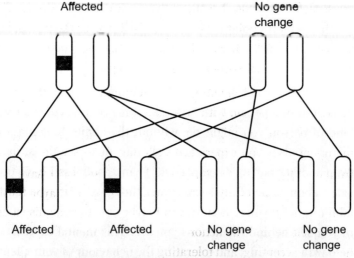

Fig. 2.5 : Dominant inheritance pattern

HD does not 'skip' generations. A child of an affected individual is at 50% risk of inheriting HD. Therefore, the implications for the whole family of a person being diagnosed with HD, are enormous.

The experience of one husband of a lady with HD demonstrates this. 'I married Wendy having no idea that her mother would become ill, but she did. We cared for her for more than ten years as she deteriorated. She lived with us many of those years and it was so hard to deal with her uncompromising demands, and later, quite bizarre and sometimes aggressive behaviour. By the time she died, the signs of HD in my wife were very evident. I look at my two young children and wonder if one or both of them will develop the same disease. Of course my concern is for them, but also, if I'm honest, I resent the fact that I unwittingly took on a caring role for each generation and devoted my entire life from the moment I got married. I wouldn't change it, but it's a daunting prospect.'

The human body is made up of many millions of cells. Most cells have 23 pairs of chromosomes. Chromosomes contain many genes. All genes are made up of sequences of chemicals. There are

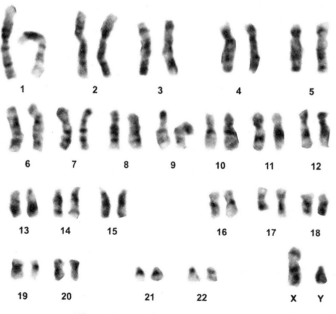

Fig. 2.6 : 23 pairs of chromosomes

four of these, represented by the letters A, C, G and T. HD is caused by a fault in a gene on chromosome 4, a gene that we all have and is necessary for life. The sequence in this gene is CAGCAGCAG... repeated. In most of us, the sequence CAG tends to be repeated perhaps 15–20 times or somewhere near. In people with HD, the CAG sequence occurs 36 times or more. Sometimes even many more than this. The number of repeats does not predict the onset of disease, but overall there is a trend associating a greater number of repeats with earlier onset.

A genetic test has been available since 1993. Most people on learning about the possibility of a genetic test for HD, think it's a very good idea for people at risk to have one. It can enable informed choices about the future. Whether to marry or have children for example. It can also enable people to adjust and make practical plans for their own care.

But when faced with the reality of deciding whether to be tested or not, good counselling will help to consider many potential problems as well as potential benefits. For example, could the person really cope emotionally knowing the outcome? What will the implications be for life insurance or a mortgage? If a pregnant woman whose partner, say, is at risk, and does not wish to know his HD status, wishes to have her unborn child tested, a positive result would tell the partner that he is positive also. How will the couple deal with this, and does the male partner have the right not to allow his child tested, to keep his own status unknown? These issues are explored further in the section on 'Big Decisions' under the heading 'tricky ethics'.

There are many more potentially difficult issues raised by the prospect of genetic testing. Some people find coping with a negative result psychologically harmful. Feelings of guilt can arise over being the one in the family who got away with it.

All of these issues and others need to be addressed with the person couple or family as appropriate, with the help of an experienced genetics counsellor before testing is undertaken. The Huntington's Disease Association Family Advisor can help to make sure people affected by HD have this support. See the contact details at the back of the book.

While Alois Alzheimer who is discussed in the next section- is credited with describing the pathophysiology within the brains of people with HD, it was a GP from East Hampton, New York who provided the first clear and precise account of the condition's clinical presentation and by whose name it became known. George Huntington was only 22, just one year after 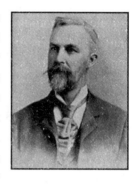 graduating from medical school when he published his report in 1872.

Since childhood he had accompanied his grandfather and his father, both doctors, on their rounds. Both had made observations of families affected by a hereditary form of chorea and George Huntington drew from these and his own observations also to compile his impressive, concise work that was to be his only research paper.

As with the other conditions outlined in these sections, many aspects impact heavily on diagnosed individuals and their carers and other family members. Some of the most difficult problems are not confined to any one particular diagnosis and we will deal with them further on.

To my knowledge by the way, the most famous person with HD was Woody Guthrie, a folk singer/ songwriter from Okemah, Oklahoma who died in New Jersey in a state hospital in 1967.

Woody is my hero. He wrote 'This land is your land', 'Ramblin' round your city' and many other songs that were warm humorous, romantic and carried strong political messages, taking a stand for disadvantaged people. He inspired many artists such as Bob Dylan, Bruce Springsteen and Billy Bragg. In fact Woody is the father of folk and country music. He carried on writing uplifting lines when very ill and is an ambassador for families affected by HD, other neurological conditions and in fact an inspiration to people faced with any of life's hardships. He faced many and HD was only one.

How else can I help?

1. It maybe helpful to join the Huntington's Disease Association (HDA) or Scottish Huntington's Association (SHA), or other national organisations. The web site details are given at the back of the book. Local and national meetings are very informative as are the newsletters. And it can be helpful to many to know that despite having a relatively rare condition, others are facing similar experiences. You are not alone.

2. Being open is helpful. This inherited condition clearly has implications for the whole family. Hiding knowledge about the risk of HD from children in the family may seem protective, but can lead to greater problems in the long run.

3. Many of these sensitive issues are difficult to deal with and you shouldn't feel you have to face them alone. The HDA and SHA have family advisors that can be very helpful in working with you to tackle these issues and many others that you may face.

4. Ensure you have access to experts. Ask your GP to refer you to a Clinical Genetics Advisor and deal with consultants who have experience with HD.

5. The final part of this book raises issues that are of importance generally to people with neurological conditions, but they have a focus on Huntington.

6. As the condition advances, people with HD find flexible thinking difficult. We have to be ready to become more flexible. There will be less anger and frustration if the day goes the way he or she wants. Where it's possible, let it happen, don't get into a confrontation, if at all possible, though of course, that is, providing what he or she wants to do is safe, and isn't hurting others. The general message? Go with the flow.

7. Tell the Family Advisors, Social Workers, and other professionals about problems and say when you're not coping. Don't tidy up for visits and put on a show. Let them see how it really is. Accept offers of respite care: you need breaks.

8. When the time comes you can't cope at home, get help to discuss the issue of nursing care. It is bound to be a difficult and highly sensitive topic and to find a suitable nursing home.

9. It's going to be difficult and sensitive, but get help to discuss 'end of life' issues early on. The time will come when it will be helpful to know the person's wishes regarding matters such as, whether and when swallowing is difficult, when eating and drinking by mouth is no longer tolerable, feeding via a tube into the stomach will be an option. Decisions are helped by taking earlier wishes into account, but when the time comes, other factors have to be considered also. If the person died from another cause, say a heart attack, would they want to be resuscitated? Would he or she want to donate his or her brain for research or education if there was an opportunity at the time of death?

These are clearly only a few points, but the involvement with experienced professionals will help you deal with other issues as they come up.

Alzheimer's Disease

There are many types of dementia; over 100 according to the Alzheimer's Society (2009) and the most common are Alzheimer's disease (accounting for over half cases), multi-infarct or vascular dementia, and Lewy body dementia. These last two will be discussed further on.

The prevalence of dementia increases with age. It affects around 5-8% of people over 65; around 15-20% over 75, and more than 25% (some estimates up to 50%) of people aged over 85. But if you work in a care setting specializing in this area, you will no doubt encounter much younger people with Alzheimer type dementia, perhaps in their early 50s or even younger.

Alois Alzheimer was an exceptional psychology and neuroscience expert from Germany, whose work on the pathology of mental illness, arteriosclerosis within the brain and Huntington's disease led the world to greater understanding. He was a great collaborator and never wrote a book of his own.

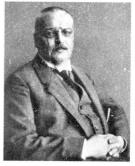

In 1901 he became interested in a patient showing signs of dementia that had tended to be associated with old age 'senile dementia.' But this lady, Mrs Auguste Deter was only 51. She died 5 years later and Alois arranged for her brain and notes to go to Munich where he was working. With two Italian colleagues he identified the amyloid plaques and neurofibriliary tangles that are briefly outlined above in the section on neurons.

It was perhaps ironic that he should have such an interest in problems associated with memory, attention and concentration, because his students are reported to claim that he would light up a cigar and place it beside a student while discussing what could be seen down the microscope; then move to the next student and do the same, eventually leaving the room with a dozen burning cigars beside students, un-smoked. However, this no doubt was an example of the difference between a disease process and absent mindedness brought about by thinking so deeply about so much.

And that's why we shouldn't start to worry when we get upstairs and wonder what we went for, or can't find the car keys, or get to the car park and have to walk about pressing the remote key until we see flashing orange lights. It happens to all of us when we are busy and pre-occupied... or not busy at all and bored. The mind playing up doesn't mean that the brain is deteriorating. So what's the difference? It is important because having established that we shouldn't panic because of some memory, attention or concentration slips. It is nevertheless important that signs of dementia are picked up early, as early intervention can slow the effects of the disease. It also allows families the opportunity to come to terms, and to seek advice

The following signs may indicate dementia (but could have other, sometimes treatable causes):

- *A profound loss of memory for recent events*
- *Losing things, getting lost in a familiar territory, and forgetting arrangements*

regarding preparing to deal with likely situations before they occur.

The 'plaques' and 'tangles' referred to in the section on neurons develop in the brain in Alzheimer's disease, killing off the cells throughout the cerebral cortex and some 'subcortical' (deeper) regions. The areas affected become grossly atrophied—that is, so many cells die that the brain shrinks, with the sulci—the natural spaces between folds of the cortex and the ventricles—those spaces filled with cerebro-spinal fluid, becoming much larger, in proportion to the decreasing matter of the brain.

- *Difficulty with abstract thinking; things maybe taken very literally, including light remarks and jokes*

- *Trouble with managing finances, making plans, following the plot of a film or a book, making a meal and so on*

- *Mixing up names of people and struggling to name common items. Maybe getting around it by saying 'where did I put my..er..oh the writing thing'.*

- *Acting impulsively, or inappropriately out of character. Perhaps arriving for a meal in a nightgown*

Notably, the parietal, temporal and frontal lobes of the cortex and the cingulated gyrus, an area that wraps around the corpus callosum, are affected. Do you recall that the corpus collossum is the sort of bridge between the two halves of the brain? The cingulate gyrus has a lot to do with forming emotions (it is part of the limbic system) and with learning and memory. Also, it is involved in controlling inappropriate 'unconscious priming'. When we encounter experiences, the next time we encounter something that partly resembles the first experience, we are 'primed' to know what to expect.

So, if I drew a part picture, and you couldn't identify it then I added more, until you knew what it represented. The next time you saw the small part of the drawing, you might have a better chance of identifying it. You would have been primed. We do this all the time, without thinking about it. When my eyes tell me that I can see a desk with the top half of a person above it, I'm able to assume unconsciously that there's a whole person, and the desk is blocking the view of the other half. If control of making links between guesses that we make all the time on this basis were impaired, we maybe tricked into perceiving the world around us inappropriately.

The signs that something is wrong, rather than forgetfulness due to a hectic agenda are subtle and individual. But people around the affected person tend to know that there's a problem. I did meet an acquaintance some time back who told me she was worried about her husband. He'd parked the car and she'd found him later walking aimlessly around the car park. 'Oh, I've done that', I said, 'some days just can't think where I left it'. She said, 'But he had no idea that he should have been looking for it'. That's the problem.

It might not have been such a problem for some very absent-minded professors, but it was a problem, because this wasn't like him. Not necessarily dementia however; there can be numerous causes of confusion, disorientation and similar problems like a urine infection that are reversible. Grief can have a similar effect as can being a mother with small children, who though lovable, at times can drive you to distraction. I hate to say, this chap did turn out to have Alzheimer's disease.

The increasing frequency with which names of people and places are forgotten is an ominous sign as are forgetting recent events and things that have been learned recently. Missing appointments when this is out of character is a sign and it is the people closest, loved ones, who tend to know first whether it is out of character. And if they think something isn't quite right, health professionals should take notice.

With progression of the disease there tends to be mood swings. Often there is good insight and with it a dreadful fear, of losing memory, losing the mind and losing 'who I am'. Gradually people with Alzheimer's tend to become withdrawn and lose confidence and find communicating difficult. As I say though, each person is affected individually, but these are typical common elements.

Some people these days with some of the problems of forgetfulness and loss of attention and memory, but not so severe as to be regarded as Alzheimer's disease, are diagnosed with 'mild cognitive impairment' or 'MCI'. According to the Alzheimer's Society (2009) only about 10 to 15 % of people who were diagnosed with MCI go on to have Alzheimer's disease.

Cause

The cause isn't known but some associated factors have been established. Age is certainly a factor; in that only a small number of people under 50 have Alzheimer's disease. In my experience of nursing young people with neurological diseases though, I have nursed a few people much younger than that with Alzheimer's type dementia. Estimates generally hold that about 1% of people over the age of 65 have Alzheimer's, whereas around half of people over 85 have it. But to say that age is an associated factor isn't to say it's a cause; many people live to be 100 without developing Alzheimer's disease.

Gender maybe a factor, as more women than men have Alzheimer's; but as women tend to live longer than men, perhaps the gender relationship is misleading. There is a relatively higher incidence among people with Down syndrome. There are certainly genetic factors being explored with genes pre-disposing people to a higher risk identified but not all people with the culprit genes develop Alzheimer's.

Head injury is associated with higher incidence and there maybe external environmental factors. Consequently, the cause is felt to be multi-factorial; that is, when a number of these risk factors coincide, the chances of developing Alzheimer's disease are much higher.

Prevention

Many of the risk factors mentioned above are set for an individual. They cannot be changed and therefore, arguably are not worth an individual being concerned with. But lifestyle can be optimised and this maybe a preventative factor. A good healthy lifestyle is worth pursuing anyway as it is associated with a reduction of heart disease, strokes, cancer and many other diagnoses. Perhaps more importantly, it can help to make life more enjoyable. The US organisation, National Institute on Aging (2009) suggest that a nutritious (balanced) diet, socially engaging activities and hobbies that are mentally stimulating can delay cognitive decline. They cite research indicating possible relationships between high blood pressure, heart disease and obesity with Alzheimer's and if this is true, clearly the same activities that prevent the former should offset the latter.

Diagnosis

The strange thing is, I've been talking about people I know or have known who have a diagnosis of Alzheimer's disease or 'AD', and yet, really that isn't possible to be so sure of. AD is only definitively confirmed after death when facts about the life course of the individual are linked with examination of the brain tissue in the post-mortem (autopsy for our American friends). But doctors are now able to make fairly accurate statements about patients who either have 'possible' or 'probable' AD. Their clinical diagnosis is based first on assessment of health, reported changes in behaviour or personality (family caregiver input is important here) and the assessment of the ability to carry out activities of living.

Biological testing, for example blood and urine tests can rule out some confounding disorders with similar symptoms. Computerised Tomography (CT) and Magnetic Resonance Imaging (MRI) scans can enable a clear view of the brain and comparative scans over time can demonstrate a loss of mass and correspondingly larger ventricles and sulci, the spaces mentioned previously. The importance of the early diagnosis for the reasons given above, to help the patient and family members, cannot be overstated.

At the same time, an MRI scan can be quite a disconcerting experience for some people with cognitive problems. Deciding whether to suggest this to someone who maybe upset by the experience is an individual consideration. Factors that will be taken into consideration may include—Is there a sufficient prospect of benefit from knowing the MRI scan result? Is the person likely to understand the need to keep still? Will he or she panic in the 'tube'? It's a harmless non-invasive process, but can make a healthy alert individual feel claustrophobic, and so can be even more daunting for someone who has some difficulty communicating or understanding what's going on.

Team consideration with family involvement is important where possible regarding making these decisions. CT scans are much easier for most patients to cope with and can detect changes that can be very useful in ruling out some diagnoses, and supporting a consultant's clinical impression. MRI scan though can offer much greater detail. As said, decisions even about whether to tell the person about the options and seek consent are individual.

The Duration of Alzheimer's Disease

This is variable and individual. Generally, the time from when obvious signs are noticeable until the person dies tends to range from around 7 to 10 years.

Treatment and Support

Just as in Parkinson's disease, drug therapy is aimed at compensating for a loss of neurons that fire the neurotransmitter dopamine across synapses, the aim of drug treatment in Alzheimer's disease is to compensate for the loss of cells that fire the neurotransmitter acetylcholine. The extent of the loss of these cells correlates with the severity of the condition (Pierre et al 2004).

The drug Donepezil whose brand name-(Aricept), Gelantimine (Reminyl) and Rivastagmine (Exelon) work by interfering with an enzyme that breaks down acetylcholine in the brain, so that more of the neurotransmitter is left at synapses to be taken up by receptors. While they all work in this way, its effectiveness varies from person to person. According to the Alzheimer's Society (2009) these drugs are effective for between 40 and 60% of people with AD leaving pretty much the same estimate for people who don't benefit from them, and they point out that for many that do, this maybe temporary. The benefits reported include reduced anxiety, greater confidence, improved memory, higher motivation levels and clarified thinking.

At the time of writing, NICE (the National Institute of Clinical Excellence) the organisation that, based on research aimed at determining the clinical and cost effectiveness of treatments, advises the UK government and provides guidelines for the National Health Service has licensed these drugs for the treatment of mild to moderate AD, and can only be given as part of NHS treatment for moderate AD.

This situation has been developing and is likely to continue changing as policy decisions become better informed by research. A further drug Memantine (Ebixa) licensed for moderately severe AD works differently from the other medicines by blocking glutamate. Too much glutamate can be released by specific cells damaged by AD, and this can cause harmful amounts of calcium to enter cells. Ebixa then reduces this damaging effect. 'Alzheimer Scotland' (2009) point out that because other drugs for dementia are licensed for mild to moderate AD, they will tend to have been discontinued by the time a patient begins to take Ebixa. However, they also indicate that some physicians feel that claims that Ebixa and Aricept together maybe more effective than either alone should be verified or ruled out by further research.

It is important to emphasise that none of these drug treatments are established as most or least effective. One drug may suit some patients better than others. Some people may experience unwanted effects. So this must be worked out for each person with the physician. Family carers play a very important role in often being able to assess the effectiveness or otherwise of a medication on symptoms that the patient may not be aware of. Of course, the patient's own perspective is vital for physicians to seek to understand and take into account before reaching conclusions about the best course of action.

As AD progresses, interventions may need to become more focussed on specific problems that make life difficult both for people who have Alzheimer's and for family members who also live with the impact of this disease. Medications, complementary therapies and lifestyle changes may need to address sleeplessness for example, or irritability and restlessness. Wandering, anxiety and depression may become problems. Again, the course of AD is individual, and ideally families should have access to the support of a multi-disciplinary team of health and social care professionals, to work with the family to find solutions.

Sometimes simple things lighten the load tremendously. A better shaped pillow, someone to come for a couple of hours in a day and take over the care from a tired spouse, or son or daughter, neighbour or friend, who is wearing out under the strain. Or maybe a respite break is needed, where the person with AD stays a week or so in a specialist care facility.

Money can be at the root of tensions between a person with AD and a family carer. Not only are there problems associated with increasing difficulty in counting cash, and calculating a household budget, but there is frustration easily turning to anger at not being able to do what used to be a simple task. There can be resentment of the carer seeming to 'take over' and make the person with AD feel foolish. Paranoia can develop with AD and the feeling can feed on suspicion that money has gone missing (miscalculated or forgotten, perhaps impulsive expenditure), and may have been stolen by the carer. The more these problems occur, the more a carer might, understandably seek to manage the money. In turn, this may feed the paranoia further, because of the perception that the carer is increasingly taking over.

Handling this without being drawn into an argument may help. Some remarks may seem spiteful and it is painful to be accused by someone you're trying to help and who seems unappreciative. Involve others, such as health professionals and a social worker early on. Especially if you are a formal carer, don't put yourself in a position where there really are questions about what has happened to some money, without the professional team being well aware of the problem and working with you to agree ways of handling the issue.

Compulsive spending can result from dementia and it can be soul destroying to be struggling to cope with helping someone who maybe depending on you in many ways including financially, and find that when the benefit payment arrives it is immediately spent on an extravagant item in which the person loses interest immediately. If you suspect that the person you care for has lost the capacity to make an informed decision, seek guidance from health professionals or a social worker. Check the principles of the Mental Capacity Act (2005) which are outlined in section D, under 'maintaining safety'. You may need to discuss the issue of Power of Attorney and the professional team members will be able to advise you on this.

It may become noticeable that the affected person becomes adept at using vague, general terms to 'bluff' keeping up with conversations. 'Oh yes, goodness gracious, isn't that something'. 'Well I never, fancy that!' They will laugh when everyone else does, as though they've got the joke, but you maybe aware that they don't have any idea what the conversation is about. You probably know that it is best not to confront this. There's no problem really if it means the person is enjoying sharing the general mood of the conversation, without knowing the detail. Let it go. But that's easy for me to say. You maybe tired, wearing down with it, and you may say something to expose the bluff, and highlight the level of dementia. Not just tired, you maybe hurting terribly to see these changes, signs of deterioration in someone you love. It's not easy to stay rational all the time.

Don't chastise yourself. It's a mistake to do it, and best to avoid. But don't blame yourself for being human. Tell your social worker you need frequent breaks to enable you to deal with these things better. Or for formal carers, perhaps in a nursing home, seek rotation among staff so that each member gets breaks from dealing with the same individual over too long a period.

Another thing people expose abruptly sometimes, to the embarrassment of the person with AD or other form of dementia is forgetting. 'I just told you that'. Again, try to avoid it, but don't beat yourself up about it when you slip. Stay cool.

In the UK, government initiatives such as the National Service Framework (NSF) for older people are aimed at setting up national standards and avoiding the patchy support that older people have tended to be provided with. As part of this effort there are specific initiatives addressing dementia. 'Living well with dementia: a National Dementia Strategy' was published by the Department of Health in February 2009 (DoH 2009) and heralds a heavy financial commitment to ensure early diagnosis and intervention and radically improve the quality of care that people with the condition receive. Proposals include the introduction of a dementia specialist into every general hospital and care home and for mental health teams to assess people with dementia. They acknowledge that this will not be easy to implement and will take time to achieve, but groups such as the Alzheimer's Society are cautiously optimistic that with their continued pressure, the government is moving in the right direction.

The general principles within the National Service Framework for Older People (DoH 2001), a ten year government plan, should make life easier for people with conditions similar to AD because of the emphasis on overcoming prejudices associated with aging; providing early intervention for 'old age conditions' accessing specialist care in emergencies; better community rehabilitation in 'intermediate care' (not a crisis and not long term); ensuring a multi- health professional assessment before placement in a care home and improving the way health professionals work with each other and with patients and carers in a partnership.

These may not be specifically aimed at people with AD, but are designed to create a culture in which the more specific initiatives can thrive. Again, groups such as the Alzheimer's Society are cautiously optimistic about progress and continue to keep pressure up, to ensure the aims become an ever-increasing reality.

How else can I help?

1. Try to adopt a style of talking to the person that doesn't confront him or her abruptly with problems to do with memory and cognition generally. So, avoid a conversation that goes: 'Did you do anything exciting yesterday?' 'No, I don't think so'. 'Yes you did, you went out with Phillip for lunch'. Try something like, 'So, I hear you went for lunch with Phillip yesterday. I bet you enjoyed that'. (If he or she wants, it can be taken as a question, but it is no problem or embarrassment if it's left as a statement).

2. Depending on the severity of the dementia, prompts might help to cue memories, and save him or her from feeling 'silly'.

3. Some family photos in the room can be helpful. Avoid photos with a great big group, say at a wedding. But if there is a wide, extended family, have separate photos for each family unit. It's clear then which children belong to which parents. An album might be good for this with a family tree. So it's easy to chat about how each family unit are related to him or her. You can have the names written under the photos.

4. An album covering important landmarks in the person's life with short statements is worth building up immediately

on admission to a nursing or residential home, and also if staying in his or her own home.

5. Carers and professionals who don't know the person's past, can then frequently go through the album with the person, and gently keep the memory pathways open and accessible. If there is enough information with pictures- in short sharp statements, there is no danger of raising questions that can't be answered and would therefore add to the pain of being aware of losing faculties.

6. One pastime I have frequently enjoyed with people who struggle with memory is asking them to describe something important from the past. It maybe a family home or a holiday location, perhaps where they met their spouse. I get a large sheet of paper, a pencil and an eraser. As they describe it, I slow them down and ask for details. I try to draw it, and get them to correct me. I say, 'I'm not too good at imagining what you're telling me. Can you help me to get it right?' It's great when they say, yes, In my case, it's after a lot of erasing... I'm hopeless at drawing.

7. One problem in a nursing home can be wandering into other people's rooms, even getting into other people's beds or putting other people's clothes on. A door handle is there to be opened! Avoid abruptly stating that they're in the wrong room, or trying the wrong door. Gentle approaches cause less distress all round, including the person whose room has been invaded. Stay cool and others will. One home I know of put up fly curtain (made up of strings of beads) in front of the doors their frequent wanderer was not intended to venture into. It worked a treat for some reason... I guess not seeing the handle, and finding the beads a bit of a nuisance to deal

with helped. But also, it made her doorway without the beads more recognisable as distinct from the others.

8. Trial and error is the key, and sharing what works with other carers.

9. Encourage getting busy, joining in with others, in tasks that aren't demanding, and won't result in a problem if they aren't done too well. Helping to tidy up and dust for example. A lady I once nursed was 101 years of age. She would help me make the beds. She would tell me, 'Come on, that will never do'. I would smile and say, 'Okay', I'll do my best. I bet I'd be stopped in many work settings now because of infection control or health and safety considerations. I would have to negotiate ways around the issues to ensure she could retain that sense of purpose, which she gained so much from. I never corrected anything or straightened any covers until she had wandered off.

10. Consider joining the Alzheimer's Society or another dementia support group. Visit their websites listed at the back of this book.

11. Download the free, and absolutely excellent guide 'Coping With Dementia' (NHS Scotland, 2009). It is available at: www.healthscotland.com/uploads/documents/9310-Coping WithDementia2009.pdf It contains a wealth of useful tips.

Lewy Body Dementia

As stated already, the most common form of dementia is Alzheimer's disease (AD), and there are said to be over 100 other types. AD accounts for over half the cases of dementia in the UK (some 700,000 people currently and increasing). Many of the problems faced by people with dementia and their families are common across the different diagnoses, and so much of what is said about AD in this book is relevant to all. There is no attempt therefore here to discuss each of the many conditions that might fit under a heading of 'dementia'. But it is worth saying a little about a couple of other conditions, at least, that are less rare than many dementia diagnoses—Lewy body dementia (LBD) here, and then *'Pick's disease'* and *'Multi- Infarct Dementia (MID)*.

Friedrich Lewy was a prominent neurologist in Zurich, and in Berlin he gained his doctorate. After working in psychiatric clinics in Munich and Breslau, he worked with our eminent friend, Alois Alzheimer in his Munich laboratory along with Hans Gerhardt Creutzfeldt and Alfons Maria Jakob, associated with the rapid onset and brutally progressive condition popularly known as *'CJD' (Creutzfeldt Jacob Disease)*. That was quite a gathering; no wonder they learned so much. Lewy, like other eminent scientists including Albert Einstein, later fled from Nazi Germany and moved to the United States.

Lewy is famous for identifying spherical masses (Lewy Bodies) in neurons that displace other components within the cells. He did this in 1912. Lewy bodies disrupt the functioning of these cells and notably interfere with the activity at the synapses of the neurotransmitters dopamine and acetylcholine. You will recall that problems with the action of these two 'chemical messengers' are associated with Parkinson's and Alzheimer's diseases respectively. So Lewy bodies do have an association with these conditions. Yet many people with Parkinson's disease never have dementia, but some do go on to develop a dementia that closely resembles LBD.

Around one person in twenty five who have dementia has LBD. It is equally distributed across genders and as generally is the case with dementia is more prevalent in people over the age of 65, and it does rarely affect younger people. The condition progresses over time similarly to AD. There are likely to be motor symptoms similar to those in Parkinson's along with cognitive effects associated with Alzheimer's disease. Memory problems tend to be less pronounced than those seen in Alzheimer's.

Planning and organising become difficult and there are problems with spatial awareness—our sort of mental map that helps us negotiate our way around the environment around us. Even though currently I can only see about a third of the room I am in, with some of what I see in my peripheral vision rather blurred, and I can't see any of what is behind me, I have a good sense of where it generally all is, and if I turn to face the door I just came in, I'd know where to expect it to be. Without visual spatial awareness, all of this would be difficult and the unpredictable, rather fragmented environment could become quite threatening.

Remember that not only people with LBD have this symptom and there are implications for the way we help people to walk around, and turn, and sit back into a chair that they cannot see. (This was referred to in the section on 'parietal lobes' earlier).

In addition to the slow movement and stiffness, tremor and expressionless face akin to PD, and the cognitive decline resembling AD, people with LBD are prone to hallucinate; typically becoming convinced of seeing people and sometimes animals that others cannot see. The level of ability tends to fluctuate with better days and not so sharp days, and sometimes the changes occur rapidly, even hourly! Day and night can become switched so that the person keeps falling asleep in the day, but at night is disturbed by restlessness, and often woken by nightmares and hallucinations. There is a tendency towards fainting and having falls.

These specific symptoms are what helps a specialist make the distinction between a diagnosis of LBD and AD. Having said that, often (especially in early stages), the alternative diagnosis is given. So, a person maybe diagnosed initially with probable AD, and later be told they have LBD. This is understandable due to similarities between the conditions. The main reason that the diagnosis is so important to make is that some drugs (neuroleptics) that might be given to calm symptoms in people with Alzheimer's disease can have side effects similar to the symptoms of Parkinson's increased muscle rigidity, slowness and so on as outlined earlier. If these drugs were given to a person who has LBD the effects could be catastrophic, exacerbating all the Parkinson-like symptoms and even potentially causing death, if muscles are no longer able to work well enough to facilitate breathing and swallowing.

Neuroleptics are generally given to treat severe episodes of mental illness and given to the right people can help reduce anxiety and improve sleeping and help solve other problems. They are often given to people with dementia in smaller doses usually for these kinds of symptoms and it is easy to see why they might be given to a person with LBD if the diagnosis were not known. Ideally, anyway, it is always better if those symptoms will respond to non-pharmaceutical (no drugs) interventions like relaxation, massage and so on as mentioned earlier. But with LBD, it is crucial to avoid the neuroleptics. These are drugs such as chlorpromazine or 'largactil'; clopenthixol or 'clopixol'; haloperidol or 'haldol' olanzapine, risperidone or trifluoperazine 'stelazine'.

Similarly, if the movement problems similar to PD are treated with Parkinson's medication, the hallucinations and confusion can be aggravated in some people with LBD, but some people do benefit and trying them does not carry as serious a risk as neuroleptics.

How else can I help?

1. Avoid resorting to drugs generally and too readily as a response to problems related to neurological disorders.

2. That isn't to suggest that drugs don't offer great benefits to many... they certainly do when used appropriately and under expert guidance, they are invaluable.

3. But clarify what the problems are. Have a look at the tips at the end of the section on Parkinson's disease. You may face different problems, though some maybe similar; but the principles to clarify the issues and coming up with innovative solutions are the same. Identify the physical, emotional, social, environmental and financial barriers.

All right, here's an example of someone in a care home with LBD, and who has become prone to falling. The carer can sit with the person and as far as is possible involve them in the analysis of the problem. This time, the 'barriers' are aspects that can be a barrier to walking around safely without falling.

Physical Barriers

Possibly the condition is worsening, and it is becoming more difficult to negotiate the room and corridors and bathrooms, because of deterioration in the senses and areas of the brain that help to maintain balance and coordination. Possibly medications prescribed, perhaps to help with sleep or nausea or anxiety for example, are causing dizziness, or disorientation, leading to the falls.

Physical Adapting

Seek a review with the consultant. Ensure you are clear about all the medications being taken, what they are for, and at which time of day they should be taken. Are they still necessary? Sometimes someone is prescribed something because they complain about that problem at that particular time. They may complain of nausea, and they carry on being given it long after the original problem has passed. All medications have the potential to cause unwanted effects.

Emotional or Psychological Barriers

If visual perception, (an important psychological aspect to remain aware of) is impaired, it is easy to misread information such as patterns on carpets, that may look like clutter to be avoided or stepped over, or 'noisy' wallpaper that makes it hard to distinguish the handrail. Think about where, precisely, falls have occurred, and if, for example, the path to the bathroom from the bed seems to be hazardous, see if there's something that would make the route clearer and more easily defined. This is where the psychological and environmental barriers overlap.

Think about the person's mood. Has it changed? Whether euphoric, or sad, the change can affect the speed the person walks at, and the amount of care the person is prepared to take. Memory problems aren't usually as pronounced as in Alzheimer type dementia, but it's nevertheless easy to forget walking aids for example, if they have been assessed as useful in falls prevention.

Social Barriers

Interactions between others could be a factor. Do people distract the person while he or she is trying to walk and negotiate the room? Remember, this is increasingly demanding attention, because of impaired visuo-spatial awareness. Are meal times appropriate and individualised? Perhaps there is a rush to get there, or maybe the dining area is too crowded? If there is a fall, do we have suitably trained people always around to administer the first aid?

Social Adapting

Educate people about avoiding distractions and especially avoiding talking to the person while not within the forward visual field. In other words, don't talk to the person if you're behind them, or even too far to one side. Wait till the person is seated. Discuss how mealtimes and other activity times can be individualised, to fit with the times of day the person finds easiest to get around. Consider separate meal sittings in a home where some people struggle with being among a lot of people.

Environmental Barriers

Walk the routes that the person tends to take, especially the ones where falls have occurred. Is the flooring level a good non-slip surface? Is it noisy and distracting, that is, could a radio be turned down a little? Are there sufficient hand rails? Be careful about walking aids by the way. There is a skill to using them effectively, and if the person hasn't got the hang of it, they may fall more frequently. Also, if the person falls with one, behind a door, especially in a small area such as a w.c., it can be very difficult to get in there and help them. Are any sharp corners on furniture avoidable along the routes? Can they be rounded off or padded?

Environmental Adapting

Make a list of any hazards you've spotted including those mentioned above. Speak to the handy person (it maybe you), or in a nursing home you may need to speak to the manager, and discuss your ideas. They should be appreciated, and usually are. I find it's in no-one's interests to have a fall occur.

Financial Barriers

Money probably stops a lot of people from getting a new fitted carpet instead of a mat, curling at the edges, or building up a low wall beside some steps to prevent a fall over the edge. Don't be afraid to ask for help. You deserve it, you need it, and it will save the NHS the cost of looking after an injured person who already had trouble enough. Seek funds actively, and put aside this feeling 'I don't like receiving charity'. You're doing a job, whether you care for the person at home, or go and visit at a care facility, perhaps occasionally bringing him or her home. Or, as a staff member or a manager in a nursing or residential home, ask for money, and don't feel bad. But be clear about what it is needed for.

Financial Adapting

At home, involve an occupational therapist in your assessment of what equipment maybe needed to avoid further falls. Also involve a social worker, for advice and help regarding how to get these items paid for. Point out that care costs will be greater if another fall occurs. In a nursing or residential home, sit with a group of staff and work out a risk assessment. Involve the person with LBD (or other neurological condition) and the family as far as possible. Get clear agreement about what is needed, and tell directors, health professionals clinical governance committees...everyone that you need the money.

Pick's Disease

The degeneration that Alois Alzheimer identified in the brains of people with the form of dementia that was eventually given his name is pretty global. That is, the whole cortex loses volume as do deeper, 'sub-cortical' (beneath the cortex) areas. Arnold Pick on the other hand in 1892 examined the brain of a man who died at the end of a progressive deteriorating dementia and found a more focussed pattern of localised cell degeneration. Like Alzheimer (and Lewy, and Creutzfeldt and Jacob) Pick was a German, born of German–Jewish parents. Okay, Germany seems to be top of the league in this book at the moment but don't forget we had Parkinson in Britain, and the American's had George Huntington. Seriously, it does seem to have been the place to pioneer in neurology. Pick was both a neurologist and psychiatrist, and after saying all that, he actually studied in Vienna. He has been described as 'modest, intelligent, principled, and dignified' (Kennard 2005). Well, he was a doctor so we would expect nothing less.

I apologise for sounding a bit light-hearted. This is an awful condition, a particularly devastating diagnosis. And the impact on families is colossal. While nursing in a professional capacity I have found a bit of humour helps and I've certainly noticed that many families, though devastated, hang on to humour for the same reason. But please don't interpret my remarks as a lack of empathy. And while on a more serious note I should add that sadly, Arnold Pick died in 1924 from septicaemia following an operation to remove bladder stones. Unlike George Huntington, who wrote the one famous, and fairly brief (but very enlightening) paper, Arnold Pick published more than 350 papers and a text book on the pathology of the nervous system.

Many authors suggest that Pick's disease, otherwise known as 'frontotemporal dementia' (the degeneration of cells occurs in the frontal and temporal lobes of the cortex) accounts for around 5% of the cases of dementia (for example, Hardin and Schooley (2002)). But it maybe more common than that. Kertesz (2006) reports that estimates range from 6-12%. Kertesz maintains that in early stages Pick's disease is under-diagnosed and Hardin and Schooley agree, indicating that it is commonly mistaken for stress, depression or Alzheimer's disease.

A problem for early diagnosis is that symptoms can be contradictory. An individual may become quiet and withdrawn while another maybe hyperactive or display erratic behaviour. As the condition progresses though the symptoms are more consistent. There are the problems you might have anticipated following our discussions so far of the effects of deterioration in the frontal cortex. Problems with planning and organising occur and there is a lack of flexible thinking, with behaviour becoming increasingly anti-social.

The person lacks motivation and is pessimistic, becomes obsessive (perhaps pre-occupied with a health problem, not necessarily real) and doesn't communicate emotionally. Family members experience the rapid loss of the person they knew, and so the caring role they find themselves adopting is tremendously hard given that their efforts may often seem unappreciated and even resented by a seemingly selfish, cold individual who has taken the place of their loved one. Yet many are able to remain aware that the affected person cannot help it and that these are the effects of the disease. Families need good structured practical, emotional and moral support.

Other effects include repetitive speech and a glazed, distant facial expression. Speech is eventually lost and there is a loss of muscle control (akinesia). 'Kinetics' refers to movement as previously discussed and 'a' in front of a word refers to 'an absence of'.

Diagnosis

Specialists will carry out a physical examination and a neurological and psychological clinical assessment. Blood tests will help to rule out other potential causes for the signs observed in the patient. Computerised Tomography (CT) and Magnetic Resonance Imaging (MRI) scans are able to detect degenerative changes in the brain.

There are striking differences in the presentation of people with Pick's disease and people developing Alzheimer's. Alzheimer's disease tends to develop insidiously as we have discussed, with subtle memory problems becoming increasingly problematic. But Pick's disease causes more serious changes in behaviour from the outset, although as mentioned above, early on these are not uniform among sufferers. Arguably it seems merciful that these people tend to appear to lack insight into their condition, but this has a huge impact on family members trying to cope and come to terms with the changes.

Alzheimer's disease is quite uncommon under the age of 65 (though I have often encountered it in much younger people) whereas generally the age of onset for people with Pick's is between 40 and 65. Survival from clinical diagnosis varies between 2 and around 17 years (some authors say 2 to 10 years). The few individuals I have been involved in nursing have been severely impaired within 2 years and survived another 6-8 years, and this seems to be fairly typical.

Cause

The cause of the changes in the brain cells is unknown, but for whatever reason, fibrous tangles of 'tau protein' called 'Pick bodies' develop in neurons in the affected lobes of the cortex (frontal and temporal) and interfere with the cells' mechanism and action. These Pick bodies are unlike the neurofibrillary tangles that we have discussed in regard to Alzheimer's disease, being straight and fibrous as opposed to coiled and paired.

Treatment

There is no specific treatment for Pick's disease, and no preventative medication so far, though clinical trials are ongoing. However, treatments targeted at specific symptoms as they occur can help to manage the most challenging aspects of the disease. Tranquilizers maybe used as may anti-depressants and behavioural therapy.

A misdiagnosis of Alzheimer's disease is unfortunate because drugs used in AD tend to aggravate aggression in people with Pick's.

Until there is an effective treatment, the management has to rely on highly skilled empathetic nursing whether at home or on a hopefully specialist-nursing facility, and social support for the individual and the family members. The particular skills involve being able to avoid a confrontation to go with the flow if appropriate or to gently change the subject or distract if it's not possible to give in to demands. These are pretty essential in caring for people with frontal lobe problems. As the Jonathan Swift quote goes — 'Don't try to reason a man out of something he didn't reason himself into. Don't argue the point when you can side-step it.' The other problems tend to be a bit more manageable if this approach is adopted.

But that's easy for me to say, I know, and no-one is suggesting there's a simple solution. As a family, you need to look after each other and be honest to yourselves if you're not coping (why should you? You weren't prepared for this). Make sure your GP, social worker, district nurses and consultant all know what you can and can't cope with, and what you need from them. Occupational health input can be very helpful and speech and language therapists also. Encouragement to take up hobbies that are not too demanding can ease boredom. Walks, music, art and photography, and jigsaw puzzles can be good; suggest it but don't push it if it isn't appreciated. Seeking respite care or nursing home admission if and when it's needed is not a failure. It's you doing your best for your loved one and for yourselves.

How else can I help?

1. This is a particularly difficult diagnosis to come to terms with. The outlook is poor and the person you care for with Pick's disease will become quite disabled fairly rapidly. Currently, death tends to occur between 2 and perhaps 10 years or longer following the diagnosis, as explained above. So this seems a good opportunity to remind carers that you need to access help. For yourself as well as the person with the neurological condition, (Pick's disease in this case) this is true regarding all the conditions we have discussed. Do join a support group. The Pick's Disease Support Group Website is listed with others at the back of the book.

2. Making the day very predictable will help. Let people know that visiting unexpectedly or doing anything that will change the routine is a bad idea.

3. Avoid any confrontation. Don't press an idea. You can come back to it later.

4. Don't argue the point. Go with the flow as far as possible, where the person you care for or your safety is not compromised.

5. Get help but insist on reliability and consistency and on someone who is prepared to be flexible and calm in all situations. You need a very experienced carer. This must be stressed to the person responsible for sending someone out to help you.

6. If the behaviour of the person becomes abusive, aggressive or intimidating do understand that it's not the person, it's the disease. But that doesn't mean you have to put up with it. Again, make sure people know when you can no longer cope.

7. Observe for what it is that triggers any angry behaviour and let people know so that they can avoid them.

8. Trial and error will help identify activities that fill the day meaningfully without resulting in stress. Some of the activities listed above are worth trying. Forget it if it isn't well received. Cross it off your list.

9. When you can't manage at home, say so. Insist. Don't say you can manage if you can't.

10. But if you do feel able to cope at home and wish to (this is true concerning all the diagnoses, not just Pick's disease), see your social worker to consider:

   i. *Respite care:* Short stays arranged for the person you are caring for at a suitable facility such as a nursing home, to give you a break. This maybe possible informally. Perhaps a family member, or a friend who can't manage continuous care, can do so for short spells.

   ii. *Day care:* Look into facilities that will have the person come once or twice a week, or maybe every weekday, for some social activity, a bath, meal and so on. You have the person back in the evening and overnight, but aren't facing 24 hour care without a break.

iii. *Meals on wheels:* Services like this in the community-perhaps help with bathing and / or dressing at home can really reduce the day's pressure.

iv. Just a point to consider about these 'help at home' services such as having a carer to bathe or dress the person. I have known carers who find that easy because they are expert in it and the person they care for is used to their way of doing it. It can be counter-productive and cause tension and aggression to allow someone else to 'help'. But these carers have tried saying, 'If you could get the children ready for school', or some other chore, 'it would help me to carry on being able to get the person with Pick's (or whatever condition) sorted out'. This idea has often been met with, 'No, sorry I'm here to help the patient, that's all, not to get children ready for school'. This is awkward inflexibility at some level. It's probably not the worker who is being awkward. It can be sorted out. Stay calm, and fix up to meet with your social worker and explain. Keep asking to see someone more in charge, if necessary, until someone is able to see sense, and give you the help that puts you in the best position to carry on caring that is in everyone's interests.

Multiple System Atrophy

Until recently the diagnosis of Multiple System Atrophy (MSA) generally wasn't made while the person was living, though increasingly it is being achieved. It is often mistaken for Parkinson's disease (PD). The patients tend to present with symptoms of Parkinsonism and Wenning et al (2004) indicate that 30% of these individuals respond well to levodopa, treatment for PD as explained earlier. Researchers are working to establish and refine methods using neuro-imaging (brain scanning) to differentiate between MSA and PD (Nicoletti et al, 2006). Despite these efforts, currently a definite diagnosis can only be made on post mortem. Physicians have to work with what clinical signs seem to indicate.

Good communication between health professionals and the patient and family is particularly important, as sometimes from a professional point of view, it makes sense to make a working diagnosis, and be flexible enough to consider other possibilities as treatment either works or is problematic. As other physicians become involved, they may use some other terminology to work with. They will understand each other but I have found that patients and their family members can lose heart and the will to carry on being concordant with health professionals over this. A particular gentleman I nursed some years back probably had MSA. Each time another name for a possible diagnosis was suggested, he became less able to consider that his consultant was trying to help him. The consultant would have been trying to act like a detective, treating the patient for one possible condition and then if the treatment didn't work, ruling out that diagnosis. Because the patient didn't understand this process, he felt that he was being treated by incompetent doctors, who kept changing their minds and disagreeing with each other. He was so infuriated, that he refused to listen to any professionals, including nurses trying to help with matters such as hygiene.

He developed skin sores, bladder retention, constipation and other problems that could have been relieved much earlier than when our team became involved. His life had become much more unhappy and uncomfortable than necessary, and many blamed him, not overtly but he sensed it and so did I. The real cause of these problems was the lack of time taken to clarify with him the meaning of and the reason for different terminology used by physicians.

There are two main clinical presentations of MSA; that is, two distinct prime sets of symptoms. 80% of people with MSA predominantly have Parkinsonian symptoms, like those we discussed in the section on Parkinson's disease. For the other 20% the main symptom is 'cerebellar ataxia'. You will recall the role of the cerebellum in coordinating movement and balance. This is a loss of that control. Sometimes these two presentations are distinguished by referring to them as MSA-P, and MSA-C, respectively. There is no clear-cut difference. The symptoms overlap, but just to clarify, this is a distinction between which of the features of the condition are most prominent.

MSA affects around 4 in 100,000 population (Vanacore 2005). It is diagnosed in men more than in women but estimates of the ratio seem to vary. Generally, it's onset begins over the age of 40, and on average between 50 and 70 according to Nicoletti et al

(2006) (though based on a Singapore study this flexible estimate seems likely to be representative of the global pattern). For most patients the prognosis is poor with an average survival of 9 years following the onset of symptoms. Frequently experienced problems include postural hypotension (blood pressure dropping when the patient stands up, causing dizziness and tendency towards falling) and urinary dysfunction. In men, erectile dysfunction happens as well. Inability to attain an erection is common.

High blood pressure when lying affects many people with MSA, and tends to be made worse by treatment to prevent the low blood pressure on standing. High blood pressure brings its own hazards leaving people prone to many serious conditions including heart disease and strokes. Vocal cord paralysis and loud harsh respiratory sound ('stridor') can be among other effects as can sleep apnoea (the tendency to cease breathing for short periods when sleeping). This can be very frightening for the person with the condition and for the carer, leaving both fearful about having a good night's sleep.

Management

The ataxia, 'clumsy' uncoordinated movement and balance problems don't tend to respond well to any treatment. Being helped with tasks that used to be easy- like washing and dressing can be humiliating and frustrating. The skill of assisting in a cheerful low key manner, avoiding taking over more of the job than necessary, and allowing time for the person to do what he or she can for him or herself is a priceless asset. I found with the fellow I mentioned above that rushing him along was a big mistake. And it had the opposite effect to that intended; that is, he took a lot longer to get dressed, wash, go to the toilet or eat a meal. If I needed to help with hooking a sock over his toes, which he was capable of pulling up the rest of the way, he would be irritated if I did more than my bit. His frustration would exacerbate his movement problems. Then he couldn't do so much, and became even more frustrated. This was like a vicious circle slowing everything down and starting the day on the wrong foot (pardon the pun).

The problem of low blood pressure when standing (known as postural hypotension) can be aided by being taught manoeuvres safely, including moving the feet up and down at the ankle; bending forward or gently marching on the spot. Patients maybe advised to avoid standing still. Crossing and then uncrossing the legs can improve circulation. With guidance increasing the salt and fluid intake can also help. Sleeping with the head tilted helps to reduce high blood pressure while lying flat will reduce the problem of postural hypotension in the morning also. It may reduce nocturia, (bed-wetting at night) and so prevent having to get up in the night, which could result in a fall if there in postural hypotension. Blood pressure can also drop too low following a meal (known as postprandial hypotension) and this can be avoided by eating smaller and more frequent meals and many recommend that drinking coffee with a meal can help.

Drug treatment aimed at improving movement problems usually involves levodopa and other medications associated with treatment for PD (see Parkinson's section). Levodopa is reportedly effective with 40-60% of people with MSA-P (more than for MSA generally). Medications can also be prescribed for postural hypotension.

How else can I help?

1. Go to the Sarah Matheson Trust website at: http://www. msaweb.co.uk/
2. In particular, go to the page on 'Frequently Asked Questions'.

There are many useful and practical tips for dealing with specific issues and problems frequently experienced by people with MSA.

3. Deal with problems that occur using a systematic approach, such as the one I've outlined earlier, (see 'how can I help?' sections in the Parkinson's and the LBD sections).

4. Tell health professionals about problems. The more honest and open you can be, the less difficult it becomes. If you're caring for a loved one at home, talk to each other about the sensitive issues about, hygiene, problems with continence, sexuality and stress on the relationship. Talk to professionals about these issues too. They have experience in these areas, and it's only embarrassing until you find the courage to raise the topic. It's usually a lot less of an issue once you begin to talk.

Motor Neuron Disease (MND)

One of the issues discussed here is life expectancy. Please do not read ahead if you do not feel ready to consider stark facts. Of course, people are individual, and what occurs to most people with a diagnosis does not definitely happen to all.

For a decision in the brain to move a muscle in the body, impulses must travel from the motor cortex of the brain, down 'upper motor neurons' (UMN) to the medulla in the brain stem or into and down the spinal cord. Then the impulse must cross the synapse with a 'lower motor neuron' (LMN) which exits the central nervous system and carries the signal to the peripheral body and fires across the synapse at the neuro-muscular junction so that the muscle contracts. Problems along the pathway affecting upper or lower motor neurons will result in problems with messages getting through to move muscles.

UMN's are a type of what are called 'first order neurons', that is, they remain within the central nervous system (CNS). You'll recall that the CNS is made up of the brain and the spinal cord. Lesions affecting UMN's result in muscle spasticity (pulled taught) and children with neuro-muscular problems due to UMN lesions are described as having **cerebral palsy**.

'Cranial nerves' exit the brain, reaching to areas such as the tongue, facial muscles, the muscles controlling the eyes and so on. Spinal nerves exit the spinal cord reaching to the rest of the body. Motor neurons within cranial and spinal nerves are the lower motor neurons. Motor neuron disease can affect upper or lower motor neurons, or both.

It is helpful to think about motor neuron disease (MND) as four broad types, outlined below, but the difference between each type is far from clear. The MND Association (2009) point out that there is a great amount of overlap in the way they affect people.

Amyotrophic Lateral Sclerosis (ALS)

This is the most common type involving upper and lower motor neurons. The muscles in the arms and legs noticeably begin to waste, and the affected person becomes increasingly weak, tending at first to trip and drop things, and soon typically become dependent on a wheelchair. Deterioration is rapid and people with ALS tend to survive only 2-5 years following the diagnosis. The great world renowned astrophysicist and cosmologist Stephen Hawking was diagnosed with ALS at the age of 22, and has since enjoyed his married life, fatherhood, and grandfatherhood while continuing to break new scientific ground. He says life before his diagnosis was never so interesting or fulfilling as it has become since. I don't know how comforting or otherwise it is to be reminded of an exception like this. It is an awful diagnosis; there's no getting away from that devastation. Almost 100% of the affected people die within 10 years. But I think what to gain from a man like Hawking, not only people with ALS but for us all, is that had he only had a year or two years left to live, he would have lived them as fully as possible. Well, he did, thinking that was all that he had done. How long he's lived is astounding, but for me that's a minor point compared to the attitude he adopted 'knowing' that his life was nearly over. None of us can say with any certainty that we have two or five years ahead of us. Many do find that to live as though we are running out of time, as though each day is a bonus, is fulfilling. And it certainly motivates people to get things done.

I do apologise for that little upbeat rant. There's probably nothing much worse than being told by someone not faced with your difficulties to look on the bright side. It's not what I meant and sorry if it's annoying. I thought that some people will surely be helped and inspired by people like Hawking even though they are exceptional.

Progressive Bulbar Palsy (PBP)

Progressive bulbar palsy (PBP) also affects both the UMN's and LMN's, and accounts for around 25% of people with MND. The term 'bulbar' refers to the medulla, that you'll recall is part of the brain stem. PBP affects the lower cranial motor nerves exiting the medulla and reaching towards areas controlling muscles that enable speech-control of the lips, tongue and palate. People typically drool and slur their words. It becomes difficult to swallow safely, and fluids aspirate into the airways. People with PBP are expected to survive only between six months and perhaps a few years.

Progressive Muscular Atrophy (PMA)

This is a much rarer form of MND and mostly affects the lower motor neurons (LMNs). The prognosis is better with most people living more than five years after being diagnosed. In the earlier days people just seem clumsy with the hands becoming very weak.

Primary Lateral Sclerosis

This is also rare and involves mostly upper motor neurons (UMNs). Weakness is in the legs particularly but there can be upper limb weakness and speech can be affected. This condition progresses in some people into ALS, but for many, the prospects for a normal life span are good.

Management

MND is a dreadful diagnosis although for some people who have strongly sensed that all is not well, there can be a strange sense of almost relief to be told what it is, and be allowed to start coming to terms with the likely prognosis. They may need psychological help and may find comfort in spiritual guidance depending on their individual philosophical outlook. They may benefit from practical help to get their affairs in order.

For those with rarer forms of MND, although fortunately the outlook generally seems more promising, there is the problem of feeling isolated, with so few affected, and little likelihood of living near someone else sharing similar experiences. It maybe frustrating to find that their GP and other health professionals they have to turn to seem to know very little about their condition. For professionals, it is worth letting a person with a rare condition know that you have little knowledge and experience of it, and that you will regard them as the expert. You have some expert knowledge that is more general and will probably be able to draw on that to help as you work with and learn from the person.

This approach tends to be less infuriating than having to deal with a professional who seems to feel threatened by the patient and carer knowing more than them about the condition, and reacting by asserting authority and failing to acknowledge his or her limitations and the expertise of patients and relatives.

Other problems that may need to be managed include pain or discomfort related to muscle cramps and spasms. Gentle relaxation techniques may help and some find gentle massage or aromatherapy by experienced and suitably trained therapists useful. Physiotherapy can be helpful in prolonging use of affected limbs. Specialist incontinence nurses, district nurses, the GP and occupational therapists maybe able to work with the patient to reduce the impact of urinary incontinence or constipation.

Speech and language therapists can help with problems related to excessive mucous, difficulty in swallowing and coughing and choking. Breathing becomes affected in the later stages. The respiratory specialist can ease the problems and help with finding ways to get more comfortable.

Whatever specific problems are faced by the patient and/or the carer, you need to make your voice heard and obtain access to the appropriate specialist. If the right help does not seem to be forthcoming (hopefully it will be without you having to ask- your GP ideally will be making sure of this) and if you are not assertive, you need to get a good advocate who will speak up for you. A relative, friend or neighbour might come to mind. Ideally not someone with an argumentative or pushy approach, but someone who you've noticed tends to get things done the way they want them, leaving everyone they deal with happy. Contact and make use of relevant charity organisations such as the Motor Neuron Disease Association (referenced at the end of the book). Tell them what it is you need and ask for help. Don't just accept a problem causing discomfort or distress to either patients or their family members.

How else can I help?

1. Go to the MND Scotland and MND Association websites. They are very helpful. See http://www.mndscotland.org.uk/index.php and http://www.mndassociation.org/

2. They carry the 'Sarah's story' campaign, which is aimed at raising awareness. The video is rather shocking and wouldn't please everyone. But it does explain pretty graphically to people without MND, what it might be like to have the diagnosis. Some family members and others involved in caring gain a lot from becoming involved in campaigns like this and joining in events to raise money for the charities. Don't get involved out of a sense of obligation though. Do it if it's something you feel like doing.

3. Learn techniques for helping with manual handling. By lifting someone with MND who is unable to stand by themselves, you could harm yourself and the person you're hoping to help. Joints become fragile and easily displaced if handled incorrectly. Involve a physiotherapist in helping you to decide what equipment you need and how to manoeuvre. Occupational therapists are helpful here too.

4. Help the person to avoid fatigue. Plan activities in advance. If going on a day out, allow time for breaks; build them into the schedule. Regular rest opportunities are important. If you think someone's idea of a trip out or other activity is too taxing, say so. Don't get swept along because it feels awkward to say what's wrong with the plan. If people want to be helpful they'll understand and won't be offended. But with good planning there's often no need to miss these opportunities.

5. Check if the person is comfortable in a chair and in bed. Soft, slidy sheets maybe more comfortable than cotton. Helping to

change position and take the pressure off bony prominences is important especially in advanced MND.

6. Tell the doctor about any reports of pain. Support limbs, the head and the neck with cushions and pillows to help give comfort, and when the weather is cold, ensure the person is wrapped up warm. Seek a tailor-made chair that is comfortable and supportive.

7. Ask the social worker to help finding funds for this. And let the support group know what equipment you require. They maybe able to help or at least may know who can. Being unable to shiver and regulate body temperature effectively, people with MND are particularly prone to becoming too cold.

Multiple Sclerosis

Because I had been nursing a lot of people who had Multiple Sclerosis (MS) who were significantly disabled by it enough to make living at home unmanageable, I began to build up a view that this was generally to be expected if the diagnosis was made. That isn't true though. Many people with MS have friends, family members and colleagues who have no idea that they do have it. Of course, I would not have got involved with those people in the facilities I worked in, providing long-term and terminal care. That accounts for my distorted perspective.

Here are two opposite extreme examples of the variation in possible MS trajectories (that is the path or course of the condition and its impact on the person).

I was at a barbecue probably about ten years ago and an acquaintance asked about my work. I wanted to get back to the topic of where the chilled beer cans were hiding, but must have mentioned nursing and people with neurological conditions. Funnily enough he said, 'I have MS'. I was amazed. I didn't know him intimately, but I had certainly bumped into him at do's like this for many years. I had never noticed anything about his posture or movement of note, and on this particular occasion he and I had played some amateur football on opposite teams. He had tackled past me which I can tell you, is no mean feat. Well, to be honest, his four year old son had managed to do that also.

'How are you affected', I asked. 'Oh, I can get a bit tired and I sometimes have spells where my vision is blurred. But the driving authority is satisfied that I'm safe to keep my licence. The spells are short and I get a warning. It seems to come on gradually, so I know when not to drive or climb up a ladder at work'. He has his own outdoor practical and physically active business. 'Sometimes I come home early feeling shattered, but it passes. I can't do the book work anymore. My wife does all that. It would strain my eyes and I've learned that if I avoid putting myself under a lot of pressure, I can get on with life really well. A lot of the time I just forget all about it'.

Ten years later, I still see that gentleman at barbecues from time to time. I can't say I see any change and he has never mentioned it again.

On the other hand, I got to be part of the team nursing Jackie, a young newly married cookery teacher. She dropped a couple of dishes in front of her class and was embarrassed at her clumsiness. Then one day as she was demonstrating how to make shepherd's pie, her legs just seemed to collapse under her and she fell with the food crashing around her. Concerned students helped her up, but she took some time out and thought that she would be fine. And she was, over the next week or so. Then pretty much the same thing happened right in front of the youngsters again. She went to her GP, who referred her to a neurologist for neurological assessment and brain scans. She was diagnosed with a (thankfully fairly rare) progressive form of MS. Within months it was becoming more difficult to manage fairly basic activities around the house, and she had to give up her job, and claim an insurance she had previously taken out covering critical illness.

Jackie's husband tried hard but as she deteriorated he found it increasingly difficult to cope, particularly as she needed assistance to wash and dress- and Jackie herself couldn't bear to have these things done by him. She wanted to think of him as her lover and husband, not as her carer and nurse. She asked to be admitted to a specialist care home about a year after those first falls. Soon she could manage very little for herself. Her food was cut for her, and later we began to soften it to make it easy to swallow. Then she could no longer do that, and she indicated that she would like a tube inserted into her stomach so that she could be sustained nutritionally without having to chew and swallow—activities that had begun to exhaust her.

A year later, two years from having her first fall, Jackie died. The end to my fear of death began with my involvement in Jackie's approach to it. So calm and accepting- living for the day, and concentrating on what could be done, rather than what can't be done. Many of the patients I've nursed through a similar process have continued to inspire me. Near the end of her life, she said to me, 'When you live for the day, it doesn't worry you that you didn't exist before you were born. And it's not a worry that I won't exist in this physical body after I die. But anyway, I will exist in the hearts and minds of those who know me and love me. And even now, that part of my existence means more to me than this part, lying here. When it was my job to teach a cookery lesson, the important thing was to do it well and with a smile. Today my job is to sit up with help, and I'll try to do that well. It doesn't matter what the job is, as long as we give our best'. In fact it seemed to some of us that the job she was doing so well was still teaching... how to approach death well, and with a smile. No, that isn't quite right. It was how to approach life!

Oh dear, after the Stephen Hawking bit in the previous section, I intended to avoid going on about inspirational people.

I'm sure it can be annoying if you're thinking, all well and good, but meanwhile back in reality, I'm having to deal with a rotten set of circumstances. I do apologise and I don't mean to play down the difficulties faced. The thing is, I appreciate that in some strange ways, really big things to deal with (as Jackie was faced) can sometimes seem easier than the drudgery of having to struggle on with a condition that doesn't quite knock you down, but is always lurking and interfering with everything.

There are differences in us all about what certain things associated with a long term neurological diagnosis would mean to us, or symbolise for us. A good friend of mine has a wheelchair. I know that to him it symbolises his independence. It's his means of getting around, being able to socialise, and play sport (he plays basket ball). Perhaps he has days when he curses the damned thing, but he certainly seems to view it as an asset mostly.

I know a lady who resents her wheelchair thoroughly. She sees that wheelchair as if it defines her and she doesn't want to be known as 'the disabled woman', 'the lady with MS', 'the wheelchair' as she tells me she has been described. That was when she went with two friends to the cinema. 'Five pounds 50p each for you two and three pound 80p for the wheelchair', the cashier had said. 'Oh, and how much if I come in with the bloody wheelchair?' came an indignant response. She told me that the cashier and her two friends had looked baffled, and seemed to decide that it must be all due to the illness.

What is Multiple Sclerosis?

According to the MS society in the UK there are about 85,000 people with this most common neurological disorder (MS Society 2009). There are reported to be around 2,500 new cases diagnosed yearly, and for most, the onset begins between the ages of 20 and

40. It is far less common in tropical climates. Scotland, where I was trained to be a nurse and first began caring for people with MS, apparently has the highest incidence in the world.

In the section on the anatomy and physiology of the nervous system earlier in this book, where the make-up of neurons, the cells of the nervous system are described, the problem at the root of MS is outlined briefly. It maybe worth having another look at it. But basically, in health, the myelin sheath that coats many axons of motor cells speeds up the transmission of signals along the length of the axon (see **Fig 1.1**). The impulse doesn't actually have to travel along in a continuous line but jumps from one of the gaps between the myelin- called 'nodes of Ranvier' to the next, therefore cutting out much of the journey.

In MS, the myelin, in patches in the Central Nervous System (CNS) (the brain and spinal cord) is destroyed, leaving the underlying wire-like nerve exposed and subject to damage. Consequently, these nerve impulses have trouble getting through, so that areas of the CNS can't communicate effectively with each other. Sometimes the message gets there but slowly and interrupted and sometimes it can be blocked altogether.

MS, sometimes called 'disseminated sclerosis' is an 'auto-immune' disease. 'Auto' refers to the self, and the term means that the person's own immune system, normally there to fight off infections and defend against disease, starts attacking the very body it should be protecting. It affects both genders but is more common in women (Debouverie 2008). The word 'sclerosis' means scars, but these multiple and widely disseminated areas of disrupted myelin are more often called plaques or lesions. The reason for the auto immune destruction of the myelin is unknown, but there are theories that implicate genetic factors, elements in the environment and infections. Perhaps all of these may play a part.

As the lesions are multiple and can appear pretty much anywhere in the central nervous system, just about any neurological symptom can occur, making it a quite unpredictable condition. Quite often, there is some physical or cognitive disability over time. Sometimes symptoms appear in an 'attack' and afterwards there seems to be complete recovery. This form of MS is known as **'Relapsing and Remitting MS'**. In another form, **'Progressive MS'**, as new symptoms appear they remain and generally deteriorate. While the outcome for individuals is unpredictable, and while rarely some people deteriorate as rapidly as Jackie, referred to above, generally the life expectancy for a person with MS is much the same as that for the wider population.

Diagnosis

Diagnosis is made by putting a number of clues or indicators together rather than through any one specific test. Some people complain of one or two short episodes of sensory or other neurological symptoms, and GPs usually advise to wait and see if they recur. If this happens referral to a neurologist is usually made. Depending on the symptoms tests to rule out other conditions with similar signs maybe carried out. An MRI scan (magnetic resonance imaging) can reveal scarring or inflammation in the myelin. A Lumbar Puncture (fluid taken from around the spinal cord) is carried out. Also neurological tests to measure the time taken for signals to travel to the brain are carried out. Typically, the eyes are stimulated by looking at a changing pattern. Electrodes taped to the head can pick up the speed of the reaction in the brain.

The neurologist may conclude a diagnosis from these tests and by considering the history reported. But it takes time to decide about the form or type of MS, because this only becomes apparent by watching the individual's trajectory or path over time. There are four generally accepted 'types' of MS, although, as said, the pattern really is individual. They are:

Types of MS

Benign MS

There maybe a few relapses (episodes of problematic symptoms) and the recovery. But neurologists wait about 15 years to ensure there are very few symptoms in that time, before they are happy to confirm this diagnosis. Even then, benign MS could develop into a more troublesome type following a further relapse after many years in some cases.

Relapsing-Remitting MS

Relapses as outlined above are followed by periods of apparent recovery and then further relapse. Sometimes the relapse lasts for weeks and other times months. Some people find that the remissions in between become less of a recovery over time and the relapses become worse. Around 80% of people with MS are thought to begin with a relapsing-remitting form. Some find that relapses tend to bring new symptoms with them.

Secondary Progressive MS

Around 50% of people with relapsing-remitting MS develop secondary progressive MS within a decade. The condition begins deteriorating steadily, rather than waiting for the next relapse. The relapses do occur, and when they are over the remissions don't follow anymore, or if they do, they do not improve symptoms in the way they used to.

Primary Progressive MS

This form of MS progressively deteriorates, without any pattern of relapsing or remission, and this deterioration continues from the outset. This is the trajectory illustrated by the account of Jackie, above.

Symptoms

As indicated the symptoms may appear and go, or maybe enduring and become progressively worse, or there may be both processes occurring simultaneously. While a wide range of symptoms are possible, most people with MS only experience a few of them. These may include problems with vision becoming blurred or seeing things in double. For most people this doesn't persist. Balance maybe affected, with feelings of vertigo, dizziness and nausea. Urinary and bowel problems are quite common and sexual dysfunction may occur.

Cognitive problems may include impaired memory, thinking and mood swings. There are quite often muscle spasms-cramps, stiffness, and speech can be affected becoming slurred and difficult to understand which in turn can lead to enormous frustration. Many people experience pain, perhaps in short bursts or continuously and it is important that this is recognised and treated, as there is a long history of doctors and other health professionals ignoring these complaints because MS was thought to be painless. Listening to what patients tell us they experience is a relatively new and an exciting concept across the board not just in neurological care. And would you know that many a time it turns out they do tend to know what they can feel!

Swallowing problems are of course serious and may result in choking or aspiration of fluids leading to conditions such as pneumonia. Fatigue is one of the most common problems. It is much more than being tired and it can be hard to get people around the person to understand that.

The acquaintance I met at the barbecue (discussed above) often described being tired, but when I enquired further, he explained that he was often embarrassed about coming home early from work. Although self-employed, he would have to make excuses to the person he was doing a job for and he felt aware that many people regarded him as 'lazy'. His wife was very understanding but when he flopped on the couch instead of helping around the house, he felt that he was trying her capacity to be empathetic, and this gave him feelings of guilt. He explained that he wasn't just tired on these occasions, but totally drained and exhausted as though his 'battery had gone flat'.

Treatment

There is no cure for MS and no one particular treatment. This is because as the symptoms affect individuals unpredictably, treatment has to be just as individualised and must aim at targeting the specific symptoms. Fatigue and mobility problems can be helped by taking regular, exercise gently. Walking is ideal. Physiotherapy may help with strengthening up the muscles. Many people claim that diet plays a part in MS, but evidence is thin. However, the healthy diet that we all ought to eat no doubt helps to manage many symptoms.

Steroids maybe prescribed for periods when symptoms are particularly troublesome, to reduce inflammation. They can have unwanted side effects so are only given as short courses. Some drugs have been credited with having a slowing effect on disease progression such as Interferon Beta-1a (Avonex or Rebif). Interferon 1b (Betaferon) and Glatirama (Copaxone) injections. The situation in the UK seems to be fairly typical regarding the approach to these interventions. They have to be prescribed by a specialist centre neurologist and will be provided by the NHS (National Health Service) only if the patient meets specific criteria set by the National Institute for Health and Clinical Excellence (NICE).

There are continuing developments in MS medications and maintaining good contact with your specialist nurse and consultant will help to make sure you are offered treatments you might be entitled to, with advice concerning their reported level of effectiveness and any potential unwanted effects. It is good to keep in touch also with organisations such as the MS society (see reference).

Baclofen is frequently used to relieve muscle spasms and stiffness and there are specific treatments for incontinence, pain, constipation and impotence. One controversial 'treatment' often gaining press attention is cannabis. It has been reported to be helpful for some individuals in improving sleep, and reducing pain. A medication called Sativex contains a cannabis extract and can be prescribed if the GP believes it will be more effective in relieving symptoms than conventional medication. However, whatever side of this fence you are on, regarding what should or shouldn't be allowed, currently in the UK, and in many countries, cannabis is illegal.

Many people with MS find relaxation, homeopathy and aromatherapy helpful but the doctor should be consulted prior to engaging in complementary therapy.

How else can I help?

1. Create a steady, reliable routine for the day
2. Make sure medicines are given at the exact prescribed time each day.

3. Ramps for wheelchairs and grab rails in the shower are examples of what can help a person with MS stay independent for longer. You maybe willing to haul the person up steps, or lift them in the shower but in doing so, you could be detracting from independence earlier than necessary and our independence is among the last things most of us are prepared to give up. That's not all of course. You probably aren't as invincible as you think, and may render the household a home for two incapacitated people. How much help will that be for the person you care for?

4. Take your time and be patient with conversations. Wait – allow a bit of silence- the answer maybe coming... processing information maybe slow...try not to cut in.

5. Keep normality going. Don't avoid public places like pubs and restaurants. If they're not properly equipped, tell them so and ask for help. They are obliged by law to be inclusive.

6. Think about joining a support group. It doesn't suit everyone, but certainly access websites such as that of the MS society (listed at the back of the book). It's a fabulous, helpful, informative resource.

Stroke

There seems to be a growing interest in changing the name of stroke to a 'brain attack'. The feeling is that the word stroke does not seem to galvanise people into action in the way that they might respond if they thought someone was having a 'heart attack'. It does seem a sensible suggestion. A heart attack happens when because of a clot blocking a coronary artery supplying the heart muscles, blood cannot get through and supply oxygen and nutrients, causing heart muscle cells to die off rapidly, impairing its ability to pump.

In very much the same way, a stroke happens when an area of the brain is starved of blood and nutrients, and consequently brain cells die off rapidly in that area. This can either be because of a clot blocking a vessel supplying that part of the brain, or because the vessel wall bursts and bleeds. Both conditions are very serious with a high fatality risk.

I do not plan to go in to great depth about stroke in this book. It is after all, a book about degenerative neurological conditions; that is, conditions that develop over time and deteriorate. Stroke is a medical emergency. It has the right name in the sense that it happens at a stroke. One second a person might possess all faculties and have full physical ability and instantly all this changes. In this sense, it doesn't fit the subject matter of this book.

But many people who survive stroke and are rehabilitated to the point where it is felt that intensive therapy is no longer appropriate are left with long term problems, often cognitive deficits and physical weakness, similar to those shared by so many of the people we have discussed so far. And so, it seems appropriate to invite people who are nursing or providing informal care for people who have had a stroke (spouses, partners, family members, friends, neighbours and so on), to consider some of the approaches we will discuss below. Certainly in our specialist care homes for young people with degenerative neurological diseases, we have cared for many people whose disability is the result of a stroke.

What is a stroke?

As indicated above, there are two main causes of a stroke. In an 'ischaemic' stroke the blood supply to an area of the brain is disrupted by a blockage in an artery. Various texts indicate that this is the cause of between 70 and 80% of strokes. The blockage can be caused by a thrombus (blood clot) that forms in the artery supplying the brain or, an 'embolism', a blood clot or air bubble or perhaps a fat globule detached from a broken bone that has formed somewhere else in the body (blood clots often form in the deep calf veins, but many strokes are caused by clots that formed in a heart chamber, as a result of a heart condition known as 'atrial fibrillation'). These clots can travel around in the blood vessels until ending up in an artery in the brain; or a blockage in the very small vessels deep in the brain.

The second main cause of a stroke is known as a 'haemorrhagic' stroke, meaning a bleed due to a vessel that supplies the brain bursting. When the vessel that bursts is within the brain, this is referred to as an 'intracerebral' haemorrhage. A 'subarachnoid' haemorrhage is a bleed in the space between the outside of the brain and the skull (check out the section earlier in the book- the 'three mothers' within the anatomy and physiology of the brain chapter).

Regardless of whether the blockage is caused by a clot or a bleed, the most common symptoms are the same. There is likely to be a loss of feeling or numbness and weakness or paralysis on one side of the body (it will be the opposite side to where the 'brain attack' - some say 'cerebral vascular accident/ incident' occurred). The face may seem to have 'dropped' on one side with an eyelid drooping, the mouth drooling with saliva and the cheek sagging. Speech maybe slurred and the person maybe struggling to find the words for what he or she wants to say.

Sight maybe affected and the person maybe disorientated and may have a severe headache. Any one or a combination of these signs occurring suddenly is significant and an ambulance should be called. The Stroke Association in the UK (2009) have recently launched a fabulous campaign that looks promisingly effective. The catchy hook is **'FAST'**, reminding people to carry out a simple Face- Arms- Speech- Test. (This test is outlined in the section on multi infarct dementia, further on). The test is gaining television and press exposure and may potentially save many lives if emergency services are contacted earlier and if government initiatives such as the National Stroke Strategy (DoH 2007) are successful in improving performance on admission in terms of early treatment by specialist stroke teams and early brain scanning.

Another event should be outlined. A **Transient Ischaemic Attack** (TIA) is sometimes known as a 'mini-stroke'. The symptoms are similar to a stroke but it only lasts for a brief period. Typically it may last for a few minutes, or sometimes a few hours. If the signs persist after 24 hours, the event is regarded as a stroke but when symptoms disappear within that time a TIA is diagnosed. A TIA is an emergency. It can be an early warning of a future stroke.

This is a brief overview of what a stroke is, and much more information is available from a range of sources including the Stroke Association (see reference).

Brief Overview of Treatment

After a stroke, people stand the best chance of recovery if they are admitted to a specialist stroke unit rather than a ward elsewhere in the hospital. Where I live in the UK, not all hospitals can provide this at the moment. A CT scan should be carried out within a few hours of the stroke occurring. If a CT scan shows no signs of bleeding an ischaemic stroke is assumed. Currently, at the time of writing, in only a minority of hospitals, a drug known as tPA can be given to 'bust' the clot. This treatment is known as 'thrombolysis'. The United States seems to have a better track record for getting this treatment to people when they need it, and in Europe the picture varies. I understand that Finland has the best record in Europe. A small but highly efficient country in this context. I'm not surprised to learn that - at neuroscience nursing international gatherings there are always progressive presentations by Finnish nurses, in my experience.

The British government is actively supporting urgent measures to increase the numbers of hospitals with suitably equipped and staffed thrombolysis units with the goal of achieving availability of this treatment anywhere in the country very soon. Drugs like aspirin prevent further build up and clumping together of 'platelets' which are sticky particles in blood involved in forming clots.

Other interventions that can be considered include the

breakdown of the clot mechanically via a catheter. Expertise is needed to maintain homeostatic control- that is, keeping factors such as blood sugar, fluids and electrolytes within normal limits, and manage skin care to avoid problems such as pressure wound development.

Haemorrhagic patients need to be evaluated for surgical intervention and treatment with anticoagulant medication to prevent further bleeding.

Rehabilitation and Care

Early involvement of a team consisting of a range of health professionals including nurses, speech and language therapists, occupational therapists, physiotherapists, psychologist and neurologist and health care assistants improve the chances of a good rehabilitation.

Good care of flaccid limbs early on can help to prevent later contractures that would impede ability. 'Contractures' are a loss of joint movement because of changes to the structure of muscles, tendons or ligaments. A good swallowing assessment can help to inform staff so that they are better able to prepare food suited to individual needs and to help appropriately with eating and drinking to avoid aspirating and risking pneumonia. Some people following stroke lose awareness of the affected side. Even when asked, for example, to draw a clock face, they may draw only half of the numbers and fail to identify that the other half is incomplete, failing to perceive any 'other half' of their world'. This is referred to as 'neglect'. The phenomenon can increase the chances of injuries such as trapping a hand in the spokes of a wheelchair without noticing, and falling over to the weak side having failed to place weight on one leg.

Speech and language therapists can also help with

communication problems, and finding ways to reduce the frustration of not understanding others and not being understood. A successful discharge home into family care or to other arrangements depends on this team working together and with other professionals such as social workers to ensure potential problems have been identified and minimised. Carer support at home needs to be ongoing. Helping to access spiritual help as appropriate according to the patient's values and beliefs maybe another important role in a holistic care plan.

Rehabilitation should begin immediately, and input should be intensive for at least a year, to maximise the potential for a full recovery.

This has, as explained, been a very brief overview, there being no attempt made to provide a comprehensive analysis of problems associated with stroke and the measures necessary to overcome them. But hopefully this overview does bring us to a point where we are ready to relate some of the discussions in the following sections on providing care for people with degenerative neurological conditions to people having experienced a stroke, as appropriate.

How else can I help?

1. Encourage acceptance of interventions such as physiotherapy, speech and language therapy and input from occupational therapists.

2. Assist with what the person can't do, but encourage independence with what he or she can do. I find that if a man, for example, can reach to shave most of his face, but needs help with one area... I will offer to do that bit first. Then it's the patient who finishes the job and gets the satisfaction of completing it. Psychologically it can be a bit demeaning if

someone else, well meaning no doubt, keeps taking over and completing the tasks.

3. Learn from the therapists what they'd like you to do in the day when helping with washing, dressing, eating and drinking, walking and getting to the toilet, that will reinforce the activities they've been teaching.

4. If the person is neglecting one side, encourage awareness of it- but be guided by professionals. At the right time, this will include speaking to the person from the neglected side, and having a locker with articles such as glasses, drinks and books on that side.

5. The Stroke Help Association web site is worth a visit, and so is the Stroke Association- see the back of the book.

Multi-Infarct (or vascular) Dementia

This term is often used to refer to what is the most common form of dementia after Alzheimer's disease. It is a dementia resulting from an impaired oxygen supply to the brain because of damage to the blood vessels that supply the brain. The damage can result from a single stroke or from a series of mini strokes, or a mixture of these types. When the cause is damage to various areas of the brain's vascular system (blood vessels) it is known as Multi-Infarct Dementia of which is explained in the next section. Please see the Glossary also at the end of the book.

The other reason for wanting to outline stroke, above, is that knowing the principle of the way it impacts on the brain makes this form of dementia: multi-infarct dementia or 'MID' easier to understand. It is the most common 'vascular' dementia type; a dementia due to problems related to the blood vessels supplying the brain. About 10 to 20% of people with a deteriorating dementia have MID, and they are usually aged between 60 (some sources say 55) and 75. Men are currently affected more than women. I say 'currently' because this maybe associated with life-style factors and of course in recent years, women's lifestyles have changed, with more taking up activities previously mostly associated with men, such as smoking.

A series of strokes gradually impair the brain's activity in the same way as described in the previous section. But usually these strokes are small. The person often seems to recover to some extent but then has the next stroke, leaving them further impaired. You could certainly tell the difference between a person with this form and someone with other forms of dementia at facilities where I have worked. On a day to day basis, you never really notice the deterioration of a person with Alzheimer's disease or Lewy body dementia. But if you went away on holiday and came back, you could notice some decline. But everybody notices when someone with MID deteriorated. We would come on duty and notice the effects of another small stroke.

The risk factors for stroke are much the same as for MID— high blood pressure and cholesterol along with having diabetes and heart disease. Smoking and a poor diet also, as I have mentioned. For MID, the most significant factor among these is high blood pressure. Of course the usual advice can help to reduce that with regular exercise, especially walking, reducing stress by relaxation, considering a job change if too high powered to allow you to unwind and so on. Of course, not having a job or sufficient income, or having a job that is not satisfying or stimulating enough is also stressful. So it's about finding the right balance for your life. And that's not easy, I know.

It pays to be observant then, when caring for an elderly person who is experiencing memory loss or other cognitive problems. It may well seem initially that these events are happening gradually, and MID maybe overlooked. Sometimes the small strokes are referred to as 'silent strokes'. They aren't noticed. But an observant carer can point out the suddenness of behavioural and other mental ability changes, which may prompt doctors to investigate further. CT and MRI scans as referred to in the 'Stroke' section, can help to diagnose MID in conjunction with a neurological examination. It maybe difficult to distinguish MID from Alzheimer's confidently, particularly as some patients might have both conditions.

The symptoms of MID may include wandering and becoming lost, difficulty managing money, or following instructions, memory problems and changes in mood. Walking may change towards fast shuffling of feet. There maybe continence problems and labile emotions – that is, switching suddenly from laughing to crying without any observable trigger. On the other hand, emotions maybe flat. There maybe extreme anxiety and confusion especially at night. Attention and concentration maybe impaired and there maybe delusions- false beliefs, for example of being somebody of great importance, or hallucinations (seeing, hearing or sensing in some other way, things that the rest of us cannot perceive).

There is a poor prognosis associated with MID and treatment is aimed at preventing further strokes. The general deterioration can lead to physical decline leading to death due to a poor resistance to infections from pneumonia, heart conditions or sometimes suddenly from another stroke.

A wrong diagnosis is unfortunate because some drugs given for other conditions can have a detrimental effect on people with MID. Some analgesics (pain killers) and anticholinergic drugs including some anti-depressants such as imipramine and amitriptyline can aggravate the confusion and the other cognitive symptoms. Sometimes when they are stopped, mental function may improve. Drugs used in the treatment of Alzheimer's disease are not helpful in MID. However, depending on the presentation, anti-psychotics may help some people in only low doses, for troublesome hallucinations or severe agitation.

How else can I help?

1. See if you can build up the caregiving team. Sadly, a lot of people are embarrassed or ashamed to discuss any form of dementia with family, friends and neighbours. But the sense of stigma eases as people learn more about dementia. And these are the most likely members of your caring team, the responsibility shouldn't all fall on one person.

2. So, look after yourself, and treat yourself when someone gives you a break. Take the opportunity!

3. Slow down when you speak with the person. This will reduce the frustration for both of you.

4. Make sure the medication prescribed is taken.

5. Look out for signs of bruising. Report this immediately to your doctor and explain the diagnosis and medication.

6. Look out for and report any deterioration in the condition, or sudden changes as occur in stroke.

Face: Can the affected person smile?

Arms: Can he or she raise both arms?

Speech: Can he or she speak clearly and understand what you say?

Test: Test all 3 if any of these problems are detected.

Time: Time is brain. Ring the emergency services immediately. In UK, it's 999; in USA its 911. Know your own country's equivalent.

PART C
SHARED ASPECTS

Problems with Orientation

You may recall that in the chapter on the anatomy of the brain, in the section on the parietal lobes, we briefly discussed their function regarding what we call 'visuo-spatial awareness'. It's that 'mental map' in respect to our surroundings—say, how a room or stairway is laid out. Also, the brain processes signals coming in from what we call **'proprioceptors'**—sensory receptors on muscles that tell us how we are positioned, which way our arms, legs and head are facing. In fact, how every part of us is placed. Putting this information about the layout of the room or environment together with our own positioning within it, we get a good sense of orientation and **navigation**.

Just try to imagine not having that function. I have often seen nursing staff trying to help someone without good visuo-spatial awareness walk towards a seat, turn and sit down. Some have a good knack of helping but some don't seem to grasp the difficulty their patient is having, and as a result they can get frustrated and misinterpret the patient's response to being subjected to an increasingly fearful situation.

We can never know what it feels like being this patient, but let's imagine that the 'map' you have of the room layout when you walk in and look around does not exist. Looking ahead, the chair can be seen, and perhaps there remains some ability to appreciate that the nurses each side of you are walking you towards it and that it is getting nearer. That in itself requires spatial awareness. When you turn around, the visual information coming in is unsteady and if you perceived exactly what the eyes see, you would have an impression of a room swinging all over the place. Normally though, the room is perceived as reliable and steady because you do not perceive the raw information that is, what your eyes are actually seeing. Your brain lies to you, knowing you won't make sense of the real picture coming in via the eyes, and provides you instead with the orchestrated version.

This patient may have lost some of that security. Maybe, the room does convincingly appear to have swung off its hinges. Now imagine yourself facing the other direction. You can see ahead, but have no appreciation that anything out of sight exists. Now, the nurses are trying to coax you to sit back into the chair. But what chair? There is nothing behind you. In fact the concept of 'behind' has no meaning for you. It's a void and they're trying to get you there, out of the world you can see, fragmented though it is and into the unknown. Terrified, you grab on to the nurses' arms with all your might. Your survival instinct may cause you to hit. You have just been labelled as 'aggressive' and may now be given medication to stop you having the motivation to grab and hit.

But if you're fortunate to have a nurse each side of you who can empathise with your predicament, they will take a different tack. Working to maximise what little capacity you have for spatial awareness, they will encourage you to reach out and touch the chair while you can see it in front of you. They may try to encourage you to develop the habit of keeping your hand there as you turn, so that while your eyes don't tell you it's still there; another sense compensates. They keep their voices low and calm, and gently remind you to trust them. It is still there and they are right with you, they won't let go till you say you feel safe.

Above all, they take their time, till you test the water and satisfy yourself bit by bit that sitting back won't mean disappearing into oblivion. That is good nursing: calm, patient, reassuring. Then gently but firmly, with consent, taking each arm, placing it along the chair arms and reassuring that it is in place and similarly, planting the feet flat on the floor, confirming that they are facing the right way—all helps to make the patient feel confident and secure in the otherwise unpredictable environment.

Other areas of function in the parietal lobes include understanding numbers, and how they practically apply to real things and to concepts and also manually manipulating objects.

But, getting back to proprioception and spatial awareness, there is more than this to our orientation within our environment. We have a highly sophisticated **vestibular system** that detects and gives us a sense of orientation within our environment. This system informs our sense of balance and also of acceleration and gravity.

In the inner ear, a vestibule and three semi-circular canals are central to this sense, helping us with postural equilibrium, informing us of the position of our head and movement of the eyes. When we move, fluid within these tiny canals moves, a bit like the fluid in a carpenter's spirit level. Tiny hairs in the canals waft with the fluid movement, and we orientate ourselves within the environment based on the movement of these hairs. It is a continual feedback system where the hairs move, the body responds to compensate, the hairs move the other way, and so on, so that we consistently correct our position.

Think about when you have spun around, perhaps on a fairground or for fun as a child. When you stopped, the fluid in the canals continued to move for some time, making you think you were still spinning. As other senses told you weren't spinning anymore, you experience the room spinning instead. You may have temporarily upset this apparatus by having too much alcohol, or perhaps you've had an inner ear infection and experienced this awful dizziness. If you're not sure how awful this can be, speak to someone with menniere's disease—a condition affecting the vestibular system.

But problems with this sensory apparatus can also lead to a loss of the senses of gravity and of acceleration that we tend to take for granted. Sensing gravity orientates us so that we can feel which way we are being generally pulled down to earth. In a lift, although visually, there is no change in information coming in, you can sense if you're going up or down—that's the sense of acceleration.

I recently attended a talk by Roberta Bondar, Canada's first female astronaught and the first neuroscientist in space. This was at the **World Federation of Neuroscience Nurses Congress** in 2009, in Toronto. I feel that I should give this fabulous organization a plug, for the nurses involved in caring for people with these neurological disorders. Check it out on www. wfnn.nu. Roberta spoke about the experience in space where although the vestibular system is intact, the information it usually feeds off is not there. There is no 'up' or 'down'. Trying to sleep, when nothing such as gravity holds you down, sitting in a chair with no force holding you back into it is extremely disconcerting. During take-off and right until being in outer space, the vibration is so violent that you lose control of eye movement.

Roberta explained that these very unpleasant and confusing effects can result in persistent nausea and a helpless impression of how you relate to all that is around you. When you come back to earth, you never again take those subtle senses of gravity and acceleration for granted.

These effects can be experienced by some people with neurological disease, regardless of the specific diagnosis, if the vestibular apparatus or neurological pathways to and from it, or the brain's ability to interpret the information from it, are disrupted.

The problems maybe hard for the patient to report and explain. The person may complain of feeling dizzy, or giddy, or might say something like, 'I can't tell which way I'm leaning'. He or she maybe seen to sit in a strange posture, perhaps over to one side or might have unexplained falls. They maybe nauseous. Keep a look out for signs like this, and seek the involvement of the specialist consultant. It is very tricky to deal with and of course, medicines to help nausea for example can aggravate or even be the cause of many of these effects.

Above all, what is needed, is your empathy. Show that you realise how awful and disorientating the experience can be, and be patient, especially with helping to move around, dress and wash and so on. Avoid rushing the person, or making sudden movements. Try and keep the environment predictable and limit the number of obstacles to negotiate on frequent routes.

Muscle tone

Earlier today, I was giving some nursing students a lecture on 'searching for literature'. That's the title I was given when asked to do it, and I'm glad it wasn't 'finding literature' because as I admitted to the students, I'm a lot better at searching for what I want than finding it.

When I told them that, I got some positive reaction—a couple of sympathetic laughs, a couple of half smiles, some grimaces and at least one look of disgust at the quality of the incidental supposedly humorous remarks that started poor and got steadily worse. I mean, if you're thinking, 'I don't get it, where's the joke?' don't worry, it's not you. There's nothing much to get; that's the truth. But the thing is, I had their attention. How did I know that?

There was a reaction. Sagging heads looked up just a little more. Shoulder blades pulled back a little. Facial muscles contracted to give recognisable expressions, even if it was one of disapproval. For better or for worse, I could see that we were engaging. I've just been thinking about how difficult it might have been to continue to the end of that lecture without those subtle muscle movements demonstrating some engagement. A slightly elevated eyebrow. Minimally tightened lips. Sitting back slightly for the overview—my summing up easy ideas and leaning forward slightly at a more tricky concept.

My long suffering wife can spot a mile off when I've lost track of her account of something interesting that happened in her day. I will give the right facial expressions to show that I am still very much with it, but they become exaggerated. Doing it for effect just doesn't look quite the same as true spontaneity to a seasoned facial language expert like Sioux. Damn. 'What do you think of that?' she'll ask. 'Unbelievable' I'll reply... it's safe because it could be unbelievably good or bad. She knows though.

We're talking here about muscle tone. We discussed earlier about how the neurotransmitters fire across the neuromuscular junction and cause muscles to contract or relax. But muscles aren't in either one or the other state; not in health anyway. They are in a state somewhere between the two. Most people sit to read. So I'll take a guess that's what you're doing. Think about how you're holding your shoulders. Well, I'm sure they're not firmly braced back as tight as you can get them, or pulled up towards your ears. No, I'm sure you're fairly relaxed. But not totally. Just let those shoulders loose now. Go on, a bit more. And your face muscles. Let your jaw drop. And your cheeks sag. Not your arms and hands though, or you'll drop the book! Okay, get back to normal be comfortable.

The point is, even though you no doubt felt relaxed, you hadn't just let your muscles flop- as I say. They are held in a state of tension, somewhere appropriately between taut and flopped.

The nervous system controls this level of tension and constantly reassesses your position in the light of sensory information coming in, and re-adjusts the 'tone' of the muscles. So many people with the conditions we have been discussing with impaired central nervous control are unable to maintain this rather crucial balance.

People with **spasticity** for example, perhaps following a **stroke**, or in **dystonia** (see anatomy and physiology section) or with **Motor Neurone Disease** with an Upper Motor Neuron lesion have too much tension—a high tone or 'hypertonic'. (remember that 'hyper' is high and 'hypo' is low). While people with Parkinson's for example or people with a 'flaccid' (floppy rather than spastic) paralysis on one side following a stroke (this may change to spastic paralysis without good care of floppy limbs) maybe hypotonic (too little muscle tension).

Typically, people with advanced **Parkinson's** are described as having a 'mask-like face'. They maybe laughing on the inside at your jokes, but the face looks dead-pan, or like a poker player not giving away any reaction or emotion.

On the other hand someone with a movement disorder like chorea as seen in **Huntington's disease** has constantly changing tone, much out of voluntary control. Limbs jerk, and the face make grimacing expressions and so on.

So, before we think about how these effects impair ability to move around, it's worth considering the extent to which they can impair interaction with other people. If they're not picking up cues that the person is interested in what they say, not amused by their funny remarks and so on, conversations and consequently any potential rapport can quickly fall flat. It's worth letting people know what has happened to muscle tone, and that it doesn't mean a lack of interest or wit. We will return to this issue shortly. Problems with communicating are very serious because they can result in the complete loss of your social life, and cause you to miss out on the available help, and to receive wrong treatment and care, worsening rather than improving your situation as intended. That should justify coming back to 'communicating' after some points about the impact of changes with muscle tone control on moving around.

Assessing how people are able to move around safely, with the appropriate level of help- avoiding taking over, but protecting from harm, and giving enough help to avoid frustration, needs to be individual. *Occupational Therapists (OTs)* are very helpful in working with the patient and carer to get the environment right. They may suggest significant changes and if it's going to help you cope, it maybe worthwhile. *Social Workers* can help you to work out which funding you maybe entitled to, to make the changes possible and can help you to apply. Sometimes changes needed might be small, such as a hand rail or higher toilet seat that's easier to get onto and off or maybe just re-arranging furniture so that there are less obstacles. Whether you are an informal carer such as a spouse or other relative at home, or a professional nurse, supporting at home or caring in a specialist facility, you still need this expertise to help you make a good assessment.

Particular daily activities that you may need professional help with assessing are dressing, washing and bathing or showering, sleeping (finding the right kind of mattress, bed height, adjustability, and so on), getting to and using the toilet, mobilising around the room, house or nursing home, eating and drinking. For the last of these, input from a *Speech and Language Therapist* can be invaluable. Remember that many people with neurological conditions have good days and bad days. This is true all round but particularly the case with relapsing and remitting *Multiple Sclerosis*. (Ill-informed people might jump to the conclusion that the person is 'acting' if they appear quite disabled at times and at other times able. It can be worth thinking with the affected person, whether explaining the condition to some people who jump to conclusions otherwise, is a good idea or not).

Anyway, my point here was, assessments that happen on a good day might be misleading. Make sure the health professional knows what bad days are like. Sometimes patients feel they have to impress health professionals by doing their very best, at a level they just can't keep up once the assessment is over. It's best to try to act fairly naturally and allow the professional to see how the person normally is able to manage.

You must insist that you need this help if your GP doesn't seem to be forthcoming in arranging it for you. Contact the relevant voluntary organisation (see list at the end of the book) for further help to find out whom to get in touch with for specific types of help. Life will be so much more manageable if you get the right help.

These day to day activities are severely hampered by problems with control of muscle tone. But a moment to moment activity is also greatly disrupted. That is communicating. I promised to return to this. Many say things like '85% of communication is non-verbal'. Well, I have no idea how you could put a figure on it, but I do appreciate the point made that most of our interaction is non-verbal and depends heavily on good control of and ability to read and interpret muscle tone.

If friends, relatives, colleagues, neighbours, shop assistants, bus drivers and other acquaintances are misreading signals, they may then give off their own negative signals. They won't mean to be 'off'. It just is a kind of reaction for a lot of people. We don't realise it, but Roger Highfield (2009) points out in a fabulous article in New Scientist, drawing on research by Richard Wiseman, psychologist at the University of Hertfordshire, and Rob Jenkins, Psychologist at the University of Glasgow that we do (though we don't like to acknowledge or admit it) all tend to make sweeping judgements about people's personality and character based on the first moment we see their face.

So, if people do seem to ignore someone you're caring for with muscle tone problems or seem to 'snap' at them or give some other negative feedback, try not to escalate the situation by assuming they are unkind, or ignorant and in turn, giving them bad vibes. Cut them a bit of slack and if you smile, it may help.

Once people get to understand that this aspect of communication is impaired and they focus instead on verbal communication much more, they may begin to overlook the mixed non-verbal signals. That's good, because if the affected person is feeling low, and is losing self esteem, the bad reaction to his or her posture and facial expression will only serve to increase the problem. Added to that, slurred speech in **Huntington's** or the classic 'monotone' voice in **Parkinson's** for example, can unconsciously reinforce a prejudice view that what the person wants to say will be uninteresting.

Making sure that people around, engaged in social situations understand all this can really help the person feel better about maintaining a social life and avoid becoming withdrawn.

Carers must be aware too that being with someone who is unable to smile when you help them, or give other positive non-verbal messages, can bring you down. You need breaks to keep up a social life. Help is all around. But you must insist if it isn't forthcoming. You do need breaks and you do need to get out.

As well as being misunderstood, cognitive problems can damage a person's ability to interpret body language and facial expression. People with **Alzheimer's** disease tend to be able to easily see if a face is looking happy, puzzled, angry, or disgusted, or sad and so on. And they can usually pick up cues from that and react to them. But this ability to make those distinctions tends to be impaired in a person with **Huntington's** and the resulting inappropriate reaction can be annoying, particularly as in many ways they may seem to have a level of intelligence lacking in someone with Alzheimer's, and therefore possibly won't attract as much sympathy or empathy.

Please note that although I'm highlighting certain conditions as being good examples of certain traits and patterns of ability and behaviour, the truth is all of these conditions affect people individually and uniquely. There is a great deal of overlap between conditions, but knowing about a pattern often seen in, say, Alzheimer's, that you have noticed in a person with, say, Pick's disease, or visa-versa, may help with thinking about why it's happening.

The point really of most of this book, is that having a way of thinking about why you're seeing the behaviour you're seeing, you maybe increase your capacity to deal with it. This is not a book about what to do in certain situations, but literally about trying to become less frustrated and offended, by seemingly being taken for granted or unappreciated, or having to deal with quite inappropriate reactions through realising what is causing all this; not the person, but the disease. You knew it, but hopefully, thinking about it like this, will help you also feel it. Believe me, this need is true for professional nurses as well as for carers at home. Professionals need to remember of course that they do go home after the shift, while home carers tend to do it around the clock. No-one is suggesting it isn't done with selfless love, but likewise, no-one is suggesting that the love and selflessness isn't being tested to and often beyond the limit.

I had the cheek a little way back to suggest you cut some other people some slack. And implied that by understanding the reasons for odd, demanding, perhaps threatening behaviour at times, may help you cut the person with the neurological condition some slack. Well, perhaps more importantly, certainly just as importantly as all that, you must cut yourself some slack. If you snap, get angry, can't stand seeing the person at times, it doesn't mean you don't care for or love the person. It just shows that you're still human.

Thank goodness you haven't become a robot, doing it all without any feelings left. That can happen too. *Tell* people, friends, family, neighbours and professionals how you're doing. Tell them when you can't go on. Actually, tell them well before that.

My good friend Jimmy Pollard (2008) has a fabulous book out called 'Hurry up and wait' about caring for people with Huntington's disease. But there's a lot in there that will help carers regardless of neurological diagnosis. One point Jimmy has often made is take note of what the air steward says before take-off. 'If the cabin pressure drops, an oxygen mask will drop down. If you are accompanying a child or caring for the person next to you, put your own mask on first, then you will be in a better position to help the other person'. Look after yourself and get help when you need it.

Now, you maybe thinking, 'has all that got something to do with muscle tone?' Yes, pretty much, it has. It's something we generally take for granted until it goes wrong, and then produce quite an impact. Well there's a couple of other points to make about it too.

Some people experience *'tics'* (random contractions of muscle groups), often in the face, head or neck. They cause people to twitch, blink awkwardly and repetitively, grimace and 'smack' their lips. Vocal tics can cause people to make unpredictable sounds. About a quarter of all children at some point will experience tics but these are not usually severe, and for nearly all, it passes. And adults may experience them particularly at stressful times in life. These are called transient tics.

Many have heard of *Tourrettes* syndrome—a debilitating condition in which tics are severe. Tics that may occur in some instances with the neurological conditions we have discussed, may also come and go, or may endure, and maybe aggravated by stress. Physically, there is no direct harm except that these can interfere with eating and drinking and swallowing safely when severe. But psychologically they can cause distress and socially, they can cause people to stare, or avoid the person, adding to the pressure to become withdrawn and isolated. Talking openly about this, and allowing the person to explain how they feel about it and about the reactions of other people can help some, while others seem to fare better if the 'tics' are ignored. This is individual and is worth discussing with a specialist nurse or other professional if the issue does become a problem for the person.

Similar advice might be given regarding the potential psychological impact for some individuals of **chorea**, those dance-like movements inherent in **Huntington's disease**, or due to effects of medication for **Parkinson's disease**. For similar reasons these movements can be socially disabling, causing embarrassment if food is spilled, or people seem alarmed in public, perhaps just because they have never seen someone with a movement disorder like it.

But again, physically, for many it is not such a problem, and many feel that over-zealous treatment with medication such as tetrabenazine causes greater disability than the chorea itself. The medication may reduce involuntary, unintended movements, but also reduces voluntary movement. Maybe the person would spill some tea due to chorea when picking up a cup. But at least they can pick it up independently. Some are really helped by reducing the chorea with tetrabenazine, but many find that while they won't spill so much, they cannot pick the cup up so easily. It is often given with the intention to reduce falls. But falls are less associated with chorea (although people look so off balance and about to fall) than with other movement problems. In Huntington's for example, spasticity and rigidity are more often the cause of falls than chorea. The important thing again is to make sure any prescribing is done on an individual basis, making sure the person is clearly understood about what 'he' or 'she' perceives to be the problem.

It should be acknowledged that while some individuals do not seem to be troubled by their chorea, others feel socially disabled by it. Tetrabenazine can be very helpful to some of these individuals. As with all medications though, monitoring for unwanted effects is important. Tetrabenazine in particular can cause adverse effects in some individuals.

Dystonia

Dystonia has been mentioned previously and is potentially very disabling and sometimes painful. It involves involuntary, sometimes severe, muscle contraction causing abnormal movement and posture. When troublesome it can be treated with medication, injections of Botulinum toxin, or surgery, for example, 'deep brain stimulation in which electrodes are inserted to the basal ganglia and a current stimulates the area, often with tremendously beneficial effect.

Myoclonus

Myoclonus is another movement problem sometimes associated with neurological disorders. It involves sudden contraction of muscle groups followed by relaxation. A hiccup is an example of myoclonus in a simple form. It can occur apparently randomly or maybe initiated by something happening externally, or by trying to initiate movement. A person sitting in a chair who goes to get up, may seem to leap up; or someone who intends to speak may seem to shout suddenly. You may have experienced a form of myoclonus just as you're dropping off to sleep. I do it occasionally. I seem to be about to fall and jump to right myself. My wife has never been too chuffed about this little trait. But it's a very mild form. For some the effect throughout the day and night can be severe.

Clonazepam, a tranquiliser can help and medications normally associated with epilepsy are effective for many people. There are other medications that maybe useful and again, if it is a problem, do raise it with the doctor.

Falls

Falls have been mentioned, and you should have access to a falls assessment team. This is important with a movement disorder. It is much better to address the potential problem than to fix cuts, bruises and broken bones. An incident like this can complicate all the other issues we have thought about so far – sleeping, eating and drinking, dressing, washing and so on. Independence can be lost and with it self esteem. So do get the team in, and save it from happening, by having help to maybe adjust the environment, or clothing, or having some helpful fittings added to the home.

Judging Intellect

Be careful, that's all. Take your time deciding the level at which to pitch your conversation. I'm mostly directing this comment at people like myself- trained nurses or other people paid to care formally rather than informal carers at home who will know the person well enough.

In my first year of nursing training, I remember seeing a lady with **Motor Neuron Disease** by her hospital bed, with her head and limbs moving erratically, looking agitated. I asked her if there was something she wanted. She tried to speak but I couldn't understand. A nurse called over, 'I can't get her to take her medicine. See if you can persuade her'.

The lady seemed to be gesturing towards a brief case by the bed. I had decided, based on appearance and my ignorance of uncontrolled movement, that this lady had very little capacity to understand anything going on around her. But the case contained a 'lite writer' and a pointer that fitted to her head. With difficulty she aimed the pointer at the keys and wrote me a message explaining that she had looked at the active ingredients in the medication she'd been prescribed and knew that one ingredient should not be taken along with another medication she already takes. The doctor agreed and apologised and the prescription was changed. I'm afraid I have to admit that I had not credited her with having anywhere near the intelligence to make this observation and communicate it to me despite the physical challenge.

I spoke about the misinterpretations regarding attitudes, humour and personality related to body language impaired by the mask like PD expression, or tics and chorea; but judgements about intelligence can also be way off base, and I learned that day that they cannot be based on muscle tone problems.

Memory

We tend to think of memory as sort of film clips of the past that we can switch on in our heads. Some memories are experienced as being very like the flashbulb memories. My memory of what I was doing when John F Kennedy was shot is an example of a flashbulb memory. I was only about 7 years old and I had no idea who JFK was. But I knew something big had happened as the older members of the family gathered at the radio (TV?- I hadn't seen one). I could hear, 'He's been shot'. 'He's dead'. I could only see the backs of my family as they repeated bits the broadcaster was saying. My little clip lasts a matter of seconds. But it is incredibly vivid.

It can be a good exercise to strengthen memory and concentration and other cognitive skills once in a while, to go over a flashbulb memory, and try to expand it, (providing you don't think it's a personal incident where you maybe better off leaving it, certainly without some professional guidance). Let me test my memory. Can I see what Mum is doing or is she in the kitchen? Which door did I enter the room from? There were two in that old house. What did we do next? And so on. You may not be as old as me... if you are, can you remember JFK being shot? What about Princess Diana's tragic accident? The news came through at night. I was on night duty, sitting up with a very nice lady disabled by multiple sclerosis. When and how did you get to know about it? Can you dig out details that you haven't thought of since?

There maybe other episodes in your life that are not so public. They maybe funny, or very sad, perhaps frightening... they are likely to carry a strong emotional factor, which is the reason they are imprinted indelibly in your memory. You may have some of these going back a long way into your childhood, perhaps as young as two, and you may not be able to see what is emotional about it. I have one of being near our fire place in the morning before school. I can't think of anything special about it. It seems a mundane 'clip'. But there will be something about that morning that was emotional in some way.

People with **dementia** often retain these memories, while being unable to recall what happened a few minutes ago. Actually as we age, we all seem to experience that a bit, but this is more profound. This was discussed earlier in the section on **Alzheimer's**. But here, I wanted to emphasize the benefits of practising going over these episodes with people with memory problems. It does seem to help with delaying the destruction of memories and helps the person to retain a sense of who they are.

Generally, what we call *'episodic' memories*... those sort of 'film clips' of bits of our life don't have to be so dramatic or emotional. They are scattered around our cortex, and laid down and coded in the hippocampus (remember we discussed these areas in the anatomy and physiology chapter?). So a **stroke** or some other injury affecting the hippocampus could destroy these memories and the slow deterioration of the cortex as in *Alzheimer's, Lewy body* and other dementias could gradually disintegrate them. Why then, when there is a slow degeneration, are these memories of old still pretty intact, sometimes experienced as though they were yesterday, while very recent memories are lost?

Well, I'm afraid my answer is not all that academic or intellectual and certainly not accurate. But I find that it helps with thinking about the common phenomena.

At the end of my road is a large field and in the summer it is often full of long waving grass. I don't know much about grasses, but this stuff springs back up if you tread on it, then let go. Now, as my dear neighbour, the farmer would wish, I always stick to the footpath. Let's say I didn't. Every day for months, let's imagine I walk across that field in a straight diagonal line between my house and the stretch of a canal that I like to stand by and watch the boats. One day, when I get back, I realise I've dropped my watch; the strap must have broken. I need to find it in that field.

Well, I tell a friend that it's in a huge field and I don't know the whereabouts. He might say, 'Look, you must have entered the field from the corner nearest to your house'. That makes sense; so I go there. Immediately I can see the trodden path that I've walked down so many times. If I just follow it along, looking out for anything shiny, I stand a fair chance of seeing the watch.

But let's say I didn't go down that well-trodden path. I take a new route. I didn't start from near my house, but maybe 50 yards or so to the right. Was it 100 yards? Now once on the field I went left a bit, then the other way... As I look at the field, the grass all seems pretty even having sprung back up. It's a path that's only been trodden once and it will be hard to find again. I think that watch has had it.

If you 'take' someone to a starting point that they're familiar with to find an old, often visited memory, and trigger their journey down that well-trodden memory lane, it's going to be relatively easy. Being in Cairo in the second world war, and VE day, or further back, to playing a prank with some friends at school—the details maybe easy to find once the person is helped onto the track.

Neurologically, we're talking about neurons firing in a pattern of order that they've often rehearsed. As long as someone triggers the start of the journey, walking along is fine. In fact, the trodden path is the one comfortable place where there is safety; everything seems familiar. All around that grass looks longer and there can understandably be a real fear of getting lost among it all.

Many people like to talk about 'long term' and 'short term' memory, as though it were two different entities, working in different ways and think of the short-term area as the bit most affected by dementia. There's some truth in that, and some in what I'm saying, but although the well-worn path analogy maybe a bit simplistic, I think it goes some way to aiding our empathy. Who wants to be lost amid the ever-growing thicket of new memories to keep track of, when there's a path you know?

There is some overlapping difference in the location of short and long-term memories. Long-term ones are stored in various parts of the cortex. The hippocampus is important in laying down these memories. The temporal lobe cortex also stores 'semantic' memories—facts and meanings; but these are retrieved by the frontal cortex. When you need to recall a name, and there's a delay, you know it's there, and say, 'I'll think of it in a minute'. That's what's happening, the frontal lobe is busy accessing information from the temporal lobe.

The amazing thing I think, is that if you don't have the information there, there's none of that trying to access it. Not usually anyway. You just know what you don't know. Not like a computer searching through all the information, although fast, and saying 'no matches found'. The brain works differently and will just say, 'I don't know the name of the capital of Brunei' (unless you do). All that information going in over 40, 50, 60 years or more, and you know that that fact wasn't amongst it, without checking. Truly amazing!

Now, if you are caring for someone who seems to have lost their memory, see if you can break the problem down. I thought I had a dreadful memory as a young lad. I would be sent to the shops by my Mum for sugar and bread and come back with potatoes and marmalade. Where was the change? No idea, I must have put it down somewhere. Similarly, as an adult, I had a job selling electrical goods in a large store. I'd had a pretty stressful job before that and took this one for a while to reduce the pressure, and spend a bit of quality time with the family. But I became worried- I thought I was losing my memory.

Serving a customer, I'd say, 'Right I'll just get you one', and disappear. I would suddenly become aware that I had been staring at the mountain of cardboard boxes for some minutes. Woops, I'd 'wake up', and pick one up and take it to the customer. 'I'm so sorry madam, a bit of a delay, but here's your Iron'. 'You went out there for a kettle', she'd complain. Hmmm... was I losing the plot?? Certainly my memory was going.

But to remember something we have to steer it through four stages. Attention, rehearsal, storage and retrieval.

Attention

You may recall in the section on Alzheimer's disease, that I pointed out the importance of being able to forget or ignore any stuff is as great as being able to remember it. Our senses pick up absolutely everything, and we would no doubt go crazy if our brains paid attention to all of it, stored it and kept retrieving it, reminding us of every brick in the house wall, every word of a documentary and every face in the crowded station.

And so we need to focus attention on what is important. We have to recognise what might be important. You're no good at remembering names? You probably didn't give it a lot of attention when you were introduced. Did you stop everything else you were thinking about and say to yourself. 'Look, this will be important; focus?' If not, you had little chance, but that's not about bad memory. It's about not paying attention. Clearly, I knew I had to remember the kettle (or was it an iron?) but somehow my brain was never convinced that this was important enough to really pay attention to the conversation. I was bored. It's a great job for the right person, but I was just the wrong person.

And the shopping? I'm sure that when I was sent off, I was thinking that it meant I'd have to walk past my friend's house with my Mum's colourful bag and her purse, and could see all my hard earned street credibility slipping away. I would have heard what I had to get, but it didn't register.

Well, if you suspect that's what's happening to the person you're caring for who seems to have a memory problem, start by thinking about attention, and how you can attract it more efficiently. Are there distractions? Other things competing for a limited attention span? The radio? Songs with words are much more of a distraction than just music and fairly bland 'middle of the road' music will not compete for attention as much as something either brilliant or dreadful will. An attractive nurse? I knew there was a reason for plain comfortable uniforms.

Decide whether this is something that's likely to seem worth remembering. See if you can get that point across—'You won't want to forget this'. Get rid of the competition for attention. Now sit at the person's level and when you have eye contact, and the person looks unflustered and engaged, say it.

If you can't get attention to what you're saying, it won't be remembered. Paying attention to you isn't the same as attention to what you're saying. I recall asking for directions many years ago when I was single. A pretty girl explained. 'Up the road, turn left, to the lights…'. She had brown shoulder length hair and matching eyes and... well, you got it. All these years later, I still recall what I paid attention to. The only trouble was, it wasn't the directions. Luckily, since I've been married nothing like that ever occurred again. What do you mean, you don't believe me? That's the truth!

Rehearsal: The 'working memory'

I referred to the working memory in the section on the frontal lobes. It keeps information just for a matter of seconds, allowing us to work with it. It is widely held that this activity takes place in the frontal lobe. There are some marvellous interesting theories about this and how we apparently 'chunk' pieces of information to make it manageable. But I need to keep it simple here. Do get into it if you wish. A lot of these ideas go back to ground breaking work by Baddeley and Hitch (1974) and Miller (1956). All I need to say here is that the memory will fade and be lost unless rehearsed and then moved to other areas of the brain to be stored. It will disappear faster if the working memory has to deal with other information.

So if I tell you a phone number, you'll forget it pretty fast unless you repeat it mentally; verbalising it can reinforce or strengthen the rehearsal. If I then asked your birth date, or told you mine, you would find it harder to retain the original number. With any of the conditions we have discussed where there is frontal lobe damage, this rehearsal and then preparation to transfer to storage elsewhere will be impaired.

You could help by prolonging the rehearsal, going over it a bit more, or writing it down, so that the paper becomes the working memory replacement. Nothing is guaranteed to work. It's individual and it's trial and error.

Now, about remembering names of people you're introduced to. Repeat the name, and shake hands. Picture something bizarre that is linked to the name and will remind you of the person. Yesterday I was introduced quickly to two men, Terry and John. I quickly pictured Terry in an old fashioned nappy. Well they used to be called by that name (Terry nappies- made from Terry cloth), and I pictured him eating a famous type of chocolate orange (made by manufacturers also known by his name). The chocolate was a mess all over him and onto the nappy. I imagined he said, 'I'm going to the John' (slang where I come from for toilet). It's not perfect because if I met John alone, I wouldn't have the starting point. But if I see them together again, I'll make the association. It works for me, try it, or find your own methods.

It might give you ideas to prompt the person you care for with difficulty rehearsing memories. In an example of someone doing this, they might say, 'Oh, here's your lunch, it's a shepherd's pie. Doesn't that remind you of what we had on the holiday in Wales and remember we made that joke at the time, "I hope the shepherd doesn't mind us having his pie". There you are, shepherd's pie, lovely. That's rehearsal.

Storage

If there are problems with storage that is difficult, and then I do think we may have to accept that there's a memory problem. But I do find that it usually is there somewhere even in people quite badly impaired. It's down to making a good job of the final stage— retrieval. And when you attempt to retrieve, you can give yourself clues about how you are storing, and whether you have an efficient 'filing system'. It's those 'tip of the tongue' moments that give it away.

Coincidentally, just when I was trying to think of an example of this 'tip of the tongue' phenomenon, my wife (Sioux) interrupted my writing and said, 'Who sang that song big girls don't cry?' '10cc',

I replied, like lightening. I was proud of myself and didn't know how I'd had that information from years back so readily available. But it was wrong. 'No way' she said. I went over the tune... 'Oh yeah, that's not the hook line of the 10cc song, and probably not the title'. She wanted me to forget this wrong line of thought, but my brain wasn't going to let it go. I couldn't take on the next task with this 10cc thing unresolved.

'I'm not in love', I said. Luckily, she knew it was just a song title. 'Yeah, then there's the quiet bit in the middle... Oh... it's 'big BOYS don't cry'. Right, with that resolved it was possible to switch track, knowing that somewhere in there, there's information about the other song. And the tune came just like that. I sang the hook. 'That's right' she said, 'but who sang it?' 'It was falsetto', I said (very high, as though the singer had been castrated). Pieces of the information stored were becoming available. Not necessarily the piece I wanted—the name of the band.

Sioux said, 'People at work say it's the Fountains or the Foundations or Fleetwood Mac'. 'No, it's none of them' I said knowing it wasn't. Funny, if I don't know what it is, how do I know what it isn't? I clearly have information that I can't access consciously, but on some level that I'm not privileged to be aware of, the right answer is known. It is stored. 'I remember it was four guys... and four was significant. Yes, it's the four something... the Four Tops!' We both knew though somehow, that it wasn't quite right. We couldn't think of it. 'Wait. Wasn't it to do with mountains and valleys?'

We began talking about our new grandson, only a few days old. After five girls born to our children so far, a lovely little lad named Reuben had arrived. We discussed the home birth, and how well our daughter had done. And how proud his big sister is. What a lovely name too. Without warning I exclaimed, 'The Four

Seasons', and we both knew that was the right answer.

What exactly was going on in my head about the band's name while my conscious mind was tuned into the new baby topic, I don't know. But regarding storage, I can pick up a clue about efficiency. My wife's colleagues were somehow aware that they had stored the name according loosely to the alphabet. And they knew the rough area of location, and if they just kept going through 'bands beginning with F' they would come across it. But I had stored it semantically according to facts about the band. There were four guys in it and the word four was significant. Mind you, I don't know what mountains and valleys have to do with it There will be a connection, that's for sure.

This kind of storage is most efficient if you want to remember all about things, and think about them, how they work and so on. You remember things in a way that you can understand them and think and apply the thoughts to new situations. Alphabetic storing is fine for remembering facts but only at a fairly superficial level. Good for the kind of exams that ask for right clear answers perhaps. Not so good for exams asking for a thoughtful essay on the topic. Similarly, if you want a good 'phone a friend' contact for when you're going on a TV quiz show, it maybe important to identify someone who has a lot of knowledge. But that isn't enough. You need to look for someone who stores the relevant names and facts in an easily accessible way. Unless, you don't really want to be a millionaire.

What you find to be on the tip of your tongue when you try to retrieve something will help you to think about the way you've got your storage system organised. I have to say, usually, I'm pretty much alphabetical. This was an exception. Look, this paragraph, and lots of what I'm saying about memory, is a view. There are so many ideas and ways of thinking about it. We can't be sure who's right about a lot of it. But if we find a way to make sense of the problems faced by the people we're caring for, all well and good. If an idea I suggest sit's well, and makes sense, and is helpful, use it. Otherwise, take it with a pinch of salt, at least hopefully, it's helped you think about it.

Retrieval

There are four ways to access the information held in the long-term memory or short term and if you keep them in mind, you maybe able to help the person you're caring for who has a problem with some aspect of memory. Let's stick with the person who had shepherd's pie for lunch, and let's call her Judy, and imagine that this is someone who lately, when asked what she has had for dinner, she just seems baffled and unsure whether or not she did have any.

So, we made sure we got her attention, and when we gave it to Judy, we worked on rehearsal, as suggested a few paragraphs back. So now it's near evening.

Ah.. before we go on... Frankie Valli was the singer... that's the connection. My mind was still working on accessing that memory, unconsciously, even though my conscious mind had moved on to other topics.

Recall

If you're going to ask Judy to use recall to access the information about what she had for lunch, then you'd better understand that it's the most difficult approach. Okay, it would be something like this. 'Hi Judy, have you had lunch? What was it?' That's a tough one. There are no cues to help access the memory. You're just asking her to fetch it, unaided. It's like an exam question that goes, name the five great lakes in North America. If you find that Judy is up to it, fine, encourage her. But if she's struggling, perhaps embarrassed, perhaps guessing to try not to let you down, then you need to find an alternative more suitable approach.

Recollection

Using this approach to ask Judy to access her memory of what she had for dinner, we need to reconstruct some of the memory, so that she can continue reconstructing the rest of the information. So I could draw on the rehearsal that we did earlier. 'Hi Judy, how was the dinner?' (That helps to confirm she's had it... it doesn't mean she can't remember if you asked her straight out and she couldn't answer; it just means that by posing the stark question you have placed doubts about having had it into her mind. This way, the doubt is removed). Did it remind you of the dinner we had in Wales? You know, the dinner we joked about a man with some sheep saying you'd pinched his lunch... what's it called?

That approach is a bit like saying the five lakes can be remembered if you learn the phrase: Sam, My Hamster Eats Olives. If you have known the names of the lakes, you might recollect them with the help of this cue that gives you the first letters of each.

Recognition

You could try to help Judy access the memory of her lunch by getting her to recognise it. 'Did you have shepherd's pie today or something else?' You think that's too easy and won't stretch her enough to get her improving or at least slowing down memory loss? Okay, how about, 'Hi Judy, what was for lunch? Let me guess.. fish and chips? Spaghetti bolognaise? Shepherd's pie? Oh... 'it was shepherd's pie, oh, great stuff.'

It's like being given a multiple choice exam. Two of the following are not regarded as the 'Great lakes'. Which are they? Ontario; Erie; Champlain; Superior; Michegan, Huron; Great bear.

By the way, Champlain for a short time in 1998, became the sixth Great Lake. It didn't last, and Great Bear Lake is a very large Canadian Lake, but not counted as a Great Lake either.

Recognition is a good way to go for many people with dementia. But again, it's individual, and you need to find the approach that stretches the memory a little but not enough to defeat the person or embarrass them, and as a result, convince them that they do have a hopeless memory that's not worth spending the effort on trying to improve it. Instead, when you give the right little prompts, and the person experiences being able to access a memory thought to be lost, it can be very encouraging and rewarding giving the person hope and the incentive to carry on working on it. Mood can lift as a further result, and in turn, a cheerful optimistic mood is associated with better memory.

Relearning

'Hi Judy. I want you to try to remember with me, how you enjoyed your shepherd's pie lunch today. Can you remember me coming along at 12.30 with shepherd's pie for you? I remember that when you ate it we talked about that holiday in Wales, where we had shepherd's pie before.'

A conversation like this could happen an hour or so after lunch to stimulate the memory of it. After doing this a few times, you could see if she'll be able to say something about it with less cues. 'Hi Sarah, Judy had a good lunch earlier...tell her Judy, what you had that reminded you of Wales... what was the pie? You know with meat and potatoes...'.

The last part is asking for recollection, but it's tried after some time spent on relearning.

So, here's a little example, and you could make more up to practice your grasp of the different ways to help someone like Judy access memory.

Which shirt do you want to wear? (requires recall to answer). Do you want to wear the shirt you bought when we were out last week in town... can you remember the colour of it? Remember I had a dress of the same colour and you said they match? (Requires recollection). Do you want the blue shirt, the red shirt or the white shirt? (requires recognition- usually an easier option).

Before bath—'How about getting the blue shirt on after, here it is...'

During bath—'I bet you're going to look smart in the blue shirt we got the other day in town'.

After bath—'Now, come on, remind me which shirt it is you're going to wear now..?' (Needs relearning to remember).

Remember that so far, we've only been talking about one type of memory- **Episodic memory**. As I say, the type that goes over bits of the past, and are experienced as some sort of film clip. Of course, this is a clever trick that your brain plays on you. There are no film clips. Only patterns of neurons firing off or on. They either fire or don't. So can only be in one of two states—on or off. Millions and millions of them. And the pattern tricks you into thinking you can see the images so clearly. Well of course, when you perceived the original experience, that's all that happened then- neurons fired on or off. You perceived what you saw as images, but that's a perception. There's no real image of what you see in your head. We'll do a bit about **perception** further on. Now, you've just got to get the same pattern of on and off to repeat itself in your brain, and hey presto- episodic memory.

I find the following phenomenon very interesting. Think back to some event you were at years ago, perhaps when you were quite small. A birthday or a wedding or whatever. Try to picture who was there. What they were doing. You've been over this memory many times, briefly no doubt. But think a bit harder- can you get any more information that you didn't 'see' before? As I said, this is a good exercise for you, and for many people with early dementia, it can help to slow the effects, by strengthening relationships or connections between neurons that are there, even though many are lost.

All right, now think of someone young whom you know now, say a child. Picture that child's wedding in say, 20 years time. Can you see this person grown up? Have a good look at the face, smiling. Look around at the reception. Which people are still around, and how old do they look? Have they changed much?

If you were having a PET scan (a sophisticated scan showing patterns of activity through the brain), we would see the same areas lighting up in the same way, whether you looked back, using memory, or forward, using imagination.

In fact many scientists in this field think that memory of the past and imagination of the future are pretty much the same thing. When you looked back, did you see a complete accurate replica of what you saw the first time? I doubt it somehow. You would not have perceived and stored a whole picture. Everything was happening on the move and you collected fragments of information. When you want to retrieve them, your brain knows that all these fragments won't make much sense to you. So it puts them together in a way that seems reasonable... still maybe a bit bitsy, but at least each piece makes a bit of sense.

Although, I recall seeing the backs of people listening to the radio about the shooting of JFK, I can also see their expressions as they look at each other... and some of those shots could not have been seen from where I was standing behind them all. I have memories of clear images I never could have seen at the time. Memory isn't an accurate, passive, faithful recording. It's the piecing together of little clues to make a sensible story. Just the same as your 'memory' of the future. Think about it.

So, you'll find that someone with problems with episodic memory will have similar problems about anticipating and picturing the future. Of course, we need to do that a lot. It's how we decide and plan. Shall I take the train to London tomorrow or the car? I need to picture what would happen when I get off the train. How will I find the way from the station? I can think through and imagine a delay, then it's another hour. If I take the car, at least I've got some control. If the M25 is blocked I can get on the North Circular. But what if I can't find somewhere to park? I'm picturing different future scenarios, and comparing them to reach the best decision.

A lot of that is frontal lobe activity, but also drawing from long term memory from the hippocampus, and the temporal lobes, about what the city is like, what trains are like and so on. Damage in these areas will reduce capacity for all this function.

How can we help? Assess how much of this the person can cope with without getting anxious and agitated. Maybe you should decide the complicated stuff, and just say, 'We're going by train tomorrow'. And allow some feeling of control over simpler decisions. Will you prefer ham sandwiches or cheese? Try not to take over decisions that can be made independently, but try not to bog down with worrying choices. A choice from two clear options is usually best, once cognitive problems are noticeably impacting on episodic memory.

Still we've only discussed **episodic memory**. But it is only one aspect. Here's another below:

Procedural Memories

As a child you learned to walk. (perhaps a bit of an assumption, but if you didn't, it's just an illustration). There's a mixture of luck and judgement in it. By thrashing around you happen to nearly turn over. That felt interesting, try again. You reach for something, a rattle maybe, can't quite get it. A leg happens to kick out and you scoot along towards it. Loads of other random leg movements happened, but they were quickly forgotten. But this one is worth remembering as it got results. Bad luck in a way, if scooting along like that is really successful. Because, you might not feel the need to try other precarious ways of getting around like standing up.

Eventually, sooner or later, you're up. But a leg goes forward, you wobble, lose balance and you're down again. Next time as the leg goes forward, the opposite arm moves with it like a counterbalance... and you tighten some muscles in your upper body, and behold, you stay up a bit longer. And so on. Soon, your vestibular apparatus (the mechanisms in your inner ear) are coming into play along with the cerebellum and the rest of the brain and before you know it, there is balance and coordination as you walk along.

For a while, getting it right took a lot of concentration. The conscious activity engaged the cortex, the outer, conscious part of the brain. When the pattern of activity for walking became established, this 'memory' of how to walk was passed to deeper areas of the brain involving the basal nuclei. From then on, whenever you initiated the walking action, it all happened pretty much automatically, with the pathways in the basal nuclei making it happen. That's procedural memory. The cortex and its power to consciously think when you were learning to walk were important but now, consciousness only interjects now and then- say, to negotiate round an unexpected obstacle.

That's how it was with learning to eat. Getting the spoon accurately into the bowl of cereal and scooping some up. Holding the spoon at the correct level and moving the arm steadily aiming the spoon at your opened mouth. In goes the food, and you close the lips, chew, get the food into a bolus, and then push it up to the hard palate in the mouth not forgetting to still keep the lips closed. Now the tongue guides the food back towards the soft palate. Down to the sensitive area and triggers the swallow reflex, so that just at the right moment the airway (trachea) is shut off by your epiglottis, and the path to the stomach (oesophagus) is clear... down it goes. That bit is automatic, but you must still keep the lips closed. Ready to start the next cycle?

I'm exhausted just thinking about all that has to be done in the right order. When you learned it, it all went wrong. You opened your lips at the wrong moment and the food spilled down your face and clothes. You sensed the need to move your tongue but it's hard to know which way without being able to see it. So you pushed food out when you meant to bring it in and so on. Eventually, you pretty much got it, as long as you concentrated using your outer cortex. But then it suddenly seemed to get easy, as the basal nuclei got the procedure under wraps. The first movement of the spoon seemed to set the whole thing off and you could use the cortex to think about other stuff, while your basal nuclei took you through the actions without you thinking about it in any detail.

Cleaning your teeth, doing up shirt buttons, tying a tie, driving a car or maybe playing the piano—these were all things you and I needed to think through and repeat and learn till you 'got it'. From then on, if say, in the middle of playing a piece of Mozart that I'd learned by heart (I wish) I tried to think about the next few notes, I'd be all over the place, and would struggle to carry on. I put on a tie on most days if I'm teaching. Recently our family went to a wedding. My son asked me to show him how to do a tie up. I began demonstrating and explaining but despite doing it so often, and normally while thinking about what to take to work with me (cheese sandwiches or spam?)... this time I got completely lost.

The thing is, you can go back to doing these things consciously, using your cortex, not so much your basal nuclei, where procedural memory is stored and accessed from. But it's difficult. It takes a lot of effort and needs no distractions and total concentration.

So, when the basal nuclei deteriote due to some of the conditions we have discussed, procedural memory is impaired. So is the control of coordinated movement. Tasks that used to seem simple have to be thought about carefully, using the cortex, which is also deteriorating in many cases. Thinking about this should make it easier for us to understand these problems these people face when they try to undertake ordinary everyday procedures. No wonder we find people are fumbling around with buttons and toothbrushes. No wonder when trying to chew food and prepare to swallow, the mouth is opening at the wrong moment and it's spilling out. No wonder the tongue is pushing food out when the person meant to draw it in.

So, try to eliminate distractions and make it much easier to focus. Be cool. It will aggravate the problem if there is perceived to be a time pressure. Try not to take over when with patience the person can do it. This is all easy to say, but I know it can be frustrating to watch when you think, 'if I just took over and did it we could get on to the next thing'.

Nurses or care staff who offer respite to give the home carers a break would do well to chat these daily operations through with the patient and carer. It will be so much easier and provoke less frustration and anger if everything happens in the right order that the person is used to. Getting used to changes and other people's way of working can be way too daunting and annoying for someone who is faced with having to think through every little detail of the task.

Unconscious, Traumatic Memories

We alluded to this type of memory when discussing episodic memories. I referred to 'flashbulb' memories. It's just worth adding here that we have memories that the conscious mind is prevented from accessing. They maybe associated with high levels of emotion and while to a certain extent that makes the moment particularly memorable, on the other hand, too much emotion especially negative, may cause the brain to take control and protect the conscious mind from it. Many people who have been in a car accident for example, can tell you what happened up to a point, and after a certain point, but cannot tell you anything about what happened in between. In childhood, formative years, traumatic experiences may well be too emotional for the conscious mind to deal with and maybe buried.

Some therapies for people with psychological problems in later life may be targeted at uncovering the unconscious traumatic memories. But this can be dangerous ground and needs expert handling, as the brain may have made a good judgement in preventing the conscious mind from knowing about what it can't handle. When it is done well and appropriately, with expert support, for the right individuals it certainly seems to be extremely helpful.

A developing child of course may perceive an experience to be traumatic, when no adult nearby at the time would have thought there was anything significant to worry about. And it's what is perceived that will be recorded in the brain, rather than an external overview or rational assessment of the situation. The amygdala, a small area at the end of the limbic system in each half of the brain is involved in housing long-term emotional memories. The amount of emotion then, attached to the memory will often have more to do with emotions perceived and experienced during the time, maybe days, after the event, more than at the time of the event itself.

In some cases maybe the event will never be known, but if triggered the emotional memory may be stimulated. For reasons unknown to a person, a piece of music, the sight of rain out of the window, the smell of a particular perfume or type of soap, looking down from a height, will trigger very happy or very sad memories, or perhaps other emotions such as a consuming fear. Mechanisms keep these fears and other emotions at bay, and rationally we know the music can't be that sad. But if you lost that ability, and the emotions were allowed to the fore, you might suddenly find yourself upset one minute, and overjoyed another without knowing the reason. This kind of thing can be seen following some strokes and in people with various neurological disorders at different times.

It pays not to react very much. You might offer a tissue, but we don't have to get to the bottom of what's wrong as the person won't know. However, if sad emotions persist there is a possibility of depression and advice should be sought from the psychiatric team.

Discussions about the amygdala do tend to revolve around extreme emotions but in fairness to these almond-shaped areas deep in the brain, they are also involved in responses to much more subtle emotional expression, such as being slightly lifted by someone else's smile, or concerned by a person with a stern face. If the amygdala is damaged, we may find that the person responds inappropriately to other people's facial expressions.

Instincts

Instincts are a kind of memory built in and inherited. They protect us by making us run from a situation, or react in some other defensive or proactive way. My frontal cortex may become alert to the thought that my door may not be locked, just as I'm about to get to bed. (To be honest it's my wife who suddenly thinks of this and sends me to check!). Still, let's stick to the original scenario. My frontal cortex will send a 'worry signal' to the thalamus. The thalamus will send the signal back and this 'loop' of activity will continue.

At some point, my caudate nucleus, deep in the basal nuclei will put the dampers on this worry signal- perhaps straight away... with the thought occurring to the cortex- who's going to want to break in here anyway? Or this feeling that the matter is resolved may only occur after I've done something about the problem, such as got up and checked the door is locked. But if the caudate nucleus is not functioning well due to one of many of the conditions we've considered in this book, nothing may stop the continuous cycle. I may get up, check it's locked, head back for bed... and a few minutes later I might think, 'Wait a minute, am I sure the key was properly turned?'

I think that if you recognise yourself in this, don't panic. If that happens occasionally when you're tired and you double check, we can settle for calling you cautious. But if you're up half the night and losing sleep... often... yes, that's a problem. If it's happening to the person you're caring for (it might not be about locks- maybe about pictures not being quite straight, dirt needing to be cleaned, whatever), do discuss this with your GP and see that you get help. Sometimes subtle approaches can work. Get rid of the picture if it keeps triggering the worry signal. Go with him or her to lock the door and repeat, 'So that's it done, yes? Locked, nice and safe. So we can sleep'. Get into bed, let him or her lie down. Wait a moment or two. As she or he begins to sit up slightly say calmly, but firmly, 'Yes, it's locked, remember we both checked? Good let's sleep'. Two or three times and that might be it for the night.

However, if it's not working, there are medications which can help to reduce the associated anxiety (no, not in you, but I don't blame you for thinking it!). This kind of behaviour by the way can occur in 'Obsessive Compulsive Disorder' in people with apparently no neurological disease rather as a psychological problem.

Forgetting isn't always Bad

Just a further thought on forgetfulness. The ability of the brain to forget is underrated, no doubt due to our natural fear that when we forget, we can worry that we maybe starting to develop some sort of dementia. But the brain does an important job constantly, prioritising what should be remembered and what isn't so important. Of course, we may feel the brain got that wrong if we can't think where we put a key, or forget a name we need to know.

But if we remembered everything, we would be in trouble. Overloaded with information, we would become quite ill. There have been some interesting, unfortunate and rare cases studied in psychology, where a person has been unable to forget any details of what they've seen and heard. After passing a crowd, all the faces, what people are wearing, and what they said as they passed is remembered. We cannot cope and function well without forgetting most of the information we receive. So don't rush to worry about being a bit absent minded now and then. I described a bit earlier, how to decide if memory loss is a problem, but don't worry if you've forgotten!

Perception

Thanks to the central nervous system we are able to perceive that we exist. We can perceive beyond our own confines and are aware of the existence of others also. We perceive the environment around us, our world, and how we are orientated within it; where everything we perceive is, in relation to us, and where we are positioned in relation to it. So, without a central nervous system, I couldn't know of my own existence any more than I suppose my front door step knows it's there, being trodden on. And I couldn't know of anyone else also.

Well, as yet, I've never come across anyone with no central nervous system. But, people with the diagnoses we have discussed do have an impaired central nervous system. So they do perceive, but the perception maybe distorted and inaccurate.

The world around me might not be quite as I perceive it. But my perception is all I have, so as far as I'm concerned, what I see, hear, smell, touch and taste and experience through other senses is more to me than just an interpretation of the world... it is my world.

So if my perception presented me with a world that you kept telling me was incorrect, I may find it difficult to take your word for it and dismiss the way it seems to me.

If we could understand the way the world might look to the person we're caring for, we may understand why he or she is acting a certain way that to us seems inappropriate. It would be near impossible to really understand that though. But if we thought a bit about the way we perceive things and the kinds of ways that perception could trick people, it may improve our ability to be empathetic, patient and helpful.

Recognition of Objects

We considered recognition in the context of memory and retrieval earlier. Here, we very briefly look at recognition in the context of perceiving the world around us. If I show a child a chair and teach the child the name 'chair' that goes with it, will he or she know that another object, similar but not the same is also a chair? Well, it surprises me that children do seem to pick up that skill easily. But I don't really know how they do it. My granddaughter is four. She has seen wooden chairs with a straight back, square seat with a coloured cushioned panel in the middle, and four straight wooden legs. She's seen a range of sofas. A nice big recliner. But I don't think she ever saw a swivel seat like the one in my office till today. It's on one leg that fans out at the base and has little wheels on. The seat and back are one continuous piece. It's not the colour of any chairs I think she's seen so far. When I asked her what it was, she knew instantly- and clearly thought the question was way too easy for a big girl like her. Clearly it was.

But the other day I had asked her what a chair is. She described it as having four legs and a big bit that you sit on. So how do we recognise objects? Many people believe that the brain stores up a huge bank of reference examples, and when we see an object, we match it against features that are associated with most of the examples. If it matches, it belongs in their category, even if we have never seen anything quite like it before.

If this is correct, the matching of features must be pretty flexible. My office chair doesn't have many of the features that my granddaughter's dining chairs have. Maybe one feature can carry a lot more weight than other features. The flat cushiony part that looks like you could sit on it must override the fact that other, expected features like the four legs and the straight back weren't there, and that some features like wheels were there and shouldn't have been.

I'm not going much further. Object recognition seems to be a massive subject in psychology with a lot of clever theories, not all like the matching features idea. There are so many papers and books about it, and an example of one that demonstrates the complexity of it all is Tarr and Bulthoff (1995).

The consensus seems to be that however it all works, the process requires wide-ranging areas of the brain to work in an orchestrated way to identify an object. And we do it all day effortlessly, so that the question as to how we know a cup is a cup, to someone who hasn't really stopped and thought about it, seems a stupid one. It's just obvious.

And that's just a straight forward single object. What about walking into a restaurant never seen before and recognising the whole scene for what it is- or a view of the landscape outside? We seem to be a long way from knowing how it happens. Artificial intelligence models are able to recognise objects, but generally there must be a pretty close match of features to the previously experienced objects, so they seem a long way from what my four year old granddaughter is able to do without apparent effort.

If the brain is damaged through slow deterioration or a sudden stroke, or indeed a head injury, this smoothly orchestrated skill involving so many parts of the brain could easily become compromised and often does. The world is that bit harder to interpret, and there maybe a feeling of being lost in unfamiliar territory. It's just worth taking into account rather than feel frustrated at the person standing puzzling over everyday items. Naming things can help, and sometimes prompting gently by, say, guiding a hand. 'Here you are, your cup and there you've got the handle, that's it, take your time and enjoy your tea'. You have to assess how much of this is necessary, so that you avoid patronising someone who knows very well what it is.

It can be extremely upsetting, naturally, to see a loved one reach a point where they stand looking bewildered by everyday objects. But if you can accept the reason it is so difficult to perceive, and do a bit of cheerful prompting, often the person will get a bit more into gear, as they become less afraid of the unpredictability of it all, and reassured by your calming tone.

Recognition of Faces

The processing involved in facial recognition is different to that in object recognition. Some points about facial recognition are made in the *anatomy and physiology section*, under the heading of *'Temporal lobes'* and further on under the section on *'Huntington's disease'*, and will not be repeated here. It is worth just looking at those sections again, to help with thinking about problems that can make interpreting a facial expression in some conditions, or recognising to whom the face belongs to in others.

When the limbic system is impaired, there can be inappropriate emotions associated with the recognition of faces, and in rare circumstances if the amygdala, discussed earlier, is affected, it can result in a phenomenon sometimes known as 'imposter syndrome' where because the recognition of a loved one's face fails to trigger the appropriate positive emotions, the impaired person develops a belief that their spouse or parent or whoever, must be an imposter. This is rare as said, but illustrates how important the orchestration of different brain areas is, in recognising. More subtle problems may not be as dramatic, but can put a dreadful tension between the carer and person cared for.

Hopefully, being able to consider how this might be caused could help to reduce the annoyance a carer might feel if it seemed as though the person is being awkward on purpose.

Visuo-spatial Awareness and Visual Processing

This is a sense that enables us to make a mental map of the room or area around us and appreciate our own position and orientation within it. I gave a lecture today in a new lecture theatre. As I walked in, I tried to imagine that I did not have this sense and had to rely only on what my eyes were able to see, and interpret the visual information coming into my brain literally. It was very strange.

I could recognise the floor area I was standing on but I couldn't see whether the floor met the walls, as chairs and other furniture were in the way. I couldn't see much to reassure me that my floor area was safely suspended. I could only see in front of me so had no idea if there was anything else. When a voice came from someone not in my line of vision, it was as as though it came from nowhere, from a non-existent void. (You may say it came from behind me, but without the sense of visuo-spatial awareness, there is no concept of 'behind'. I could see a lot of shoulders with heads on, sticking up above other heads and shoulders, all disembodied.

As I moved around talking to the student's heads, they and the room were spinning all over the place making me dizzy and nauseous. As I was moving and my eyes were unsteadily going up and down with each step I took, the room looked as though it were being filmed with an unsteady hand-held video camera.

The truth is of course, I tried to do it, but I couldn't really. My occipital lobe kept processing the information so that I couldn't perceive what my eyes were literally showing me. Instead, I saw what my experience and memory and logic reasoned must make more sense—a steady room, with whole students, and a floor that is substantial and meets the walls at the corners.

Our senses give us pieces of information that don't join up. Our brain processes it all to give us 'sensible' and 'likely' experiences. And as a result the world feels for most of us relatively safe and predictable.

Picture a sadly common scenario. I referred to this in the section on **Lewy Body** Dementia and promised to come back to it. Two nurses are helping a lady named Betty with dementia towards a chair across the room. On each side of Betty the nurses both support an arm. When they get to the chair, they turn with Betty and say 'Okay Betty, sit down'. 'Come on Betty, the chair is behind you'. They start lowering Betty back and down towards the chair. But Betty's visuo-spatial awareness is severely impaired. She just has no concept of there being such a place as 'behind' her. As far as she's concerned, she's being lowered back into a void. Oblivion. Panicking, she clutches anything handy to try and claw her way back towards the perceived world. Unfortunately, the handiest things to grab at tightly are the underside of the nurses' arms.

Bruised and sore, the nurses report that Betty is becoming aggressive and request that she is prescribed something to keep her calm. The medication may further dampen her cognitive ability, and have other unwanted effects such as making her more prone to constipation.

By stimulating other senses, it's possible to help Betty to compensate for a lack of awareness of the location of the chair behind her. Talking to her calmly and reassuringly on the way to the chair about what was going to happen may help. 'See the chair Betty, that's where we're heading. When we turn it will still be there, right behind you'. 'Now we're near enough to reach and touch the chair. We've got you Betty, could you reach out and touch the chair?' 'Okay, keep touching the chair while we turn. Can you still feel it there behind you now and against the back of your legs? Take your time Betty, and when you feel ready, just gently lower yourself. We're here, and you can feel the chair. Good stuff Betty. Well done!'

Nothing works all the time and trial and error is the way. But this approach has to be better than the first one.

PART D
MORE ISSUES

Maintaining Safety

In this section, I am going to place some extracts from my previous book 'Huntington's Disease: A Nursing Guide (Smith 2005), among some other notes to raise a few more important issues. The extracts of course will mostly focus on HD, but they are relevant to people more generally with neurological disease. They are targeted at a nursing home environment, but issues may have relevance to home care too. Hopefully the extracts will help with thinking about issues that could be important to consider when making a nursing plan.

Avoiding untoward incidents, by maintaining a safe environment, I feel, is a good place to begin when coming up with a nursing or a care plan. As Florence Nightingale pointed out, 'Hopefully as nurses we will benefit our patients, but when we can't do that, we should at least ensure we do them no harm. It would be awful if someone came to harm just because they were in our care' (Nightingale, 1858).

We should begin by assessing the ability of the person we care for to maintain a safe environment independently. We need to strike a careful balance, maximising this independence, while intervening where necessary to prevent harm. This will involve taking risks, and skillfully assessing those risks to intervene appropriately without being over-protective or negligent. That really is pretty tricky.

Preventing Falls

Most of the HD clients I have met even when they have quite pronounced chorea, have a remarkable capacity to remain firmly on their own two feet. One relative who used to visit a home used to try and cover up what seemed to the staff as the early indications of the movement disorder. When sitting she would sit on her slightly fidgety hands. When she got up to walk, she would occasionally miss-step, and would look back at the carpet as if to imply that she must have tripped on some uneven pile. But I never saw her fall. The staff just ignored the miss-steps and fidgeting. I think they were right. What do you think?

On the other hand, Jack had a severe movement disorder. His arms would suddenly fly out as he walked. His trunk lurched over to the right. Just when you felt he was way past a point of no return and were sorely tempted to try and catch him, his knees dropped, lowering his centre of gravity, and he seemed to bounce back up leaning this time to the left; and so on.

Watching Jack walk was like watching a gyroscope, something I always found fascinating, seemingly defying the laws of physics. But Jack did have falls. These tended to happen mostly in the bathroom (the toilet was in there also), and outside the lift (elevator). What these two places had in common was their confined space. There just wasn't room for that correction of balance. He'd go over against the wall, but not far. He tried to correct himself by putting his hand out rather than drop his knees. Of course, his arm movements were uncoordinated. He lost balance and went over. The other factors were that in both those places he was trying to do something else other than stay upright— he was either trying to operate the lift button, or pull down his trousers and lift the toilet seat. One other situation tended to precede some of Jack's falls. That was when a staff member or someone else spoke to him, called out his name, or touched him from behind. He would try to turn on his heel to see the person, and down he would fall.

The staff were brilliant with Jack. They resisted trying to catch him. Only new staff members tended to try and do that. In moving and handling, they learned to prepare to protect falling people rather than catch them, mainly to avoid harming their own backs. But the experienced staff were braver still. They left him well alone, knowing that running up behind him or towards him could interfere with his incredible self-righting capability. If they had something to tell him, they got well within his range of vision first. And they continued to monitor Jack over time, knowing that at some point he may not find it so easy to right himself, and then a new plan of action would have to be considered.

Jack would never have made it safely down the stairs, that's for sure. So they had a combination lock put on a door at the top and bottom of the flight and encouraged Jack to use the lift, which he accepted. But then these falls kept occurring. Someone suggested taking him in a wheelchair, which he seemed to accept. But others were concerned that he was losing his independence. He didn't see the point of getting out of the chair when he got to the bottom, and in their hurry to get through the busy day, some found it easier and quicker to push him along to the dining room than try and persuade him to get out of the wheelchair and walk.

Due to these concerns about his potential loss of independence, the staff agreed with Jack to abandon the chair idea, and instead, they looked out for him heading up to the lift and made a point of running ahead to hold the button before he got there. This wasn't easy on busy shifts, but in the long term they reasoned that helping him up, patching minor cuts and bruises, going with him and the chair, were less dignified, more time consuming and less acceptable. What a great team!

They did a similar thing to resolve the problem in the bathroom. They went with him, and encouraged him to sit on the toilet with his trousers on. Then he would undo the zip while sitting, pull his trousers down and go in a sitting position. It took a while before this became a habit with Jack often losing his patience with them interfering with him just wanting to get there. When it did become a habit the staff knew that he would stick to it, and gradually they didn't have to go in with him anymore, and he regained some of his independence. Isn't that what rehabilitation is? When did you last hear that word rehabilitation in connection with a degenerative disease? But that's just what rehab is, regaining independence. There's another name for it. Nursing! Nursing is about making it possible, not taking over.

So, keep your eye on the goal—maximum independence with minimum risk. Ideally, if it's possible it can be good to choose a home with wide corridors and spacious rooms. However, you might try these ideas and find they don't work out as you would hope. You then have to try other ideas and find out what works by a process of elimination. What worked for Jack might not be any good for the person you are caring for.

Some facilities tend to encourage people to wear protective hats, and elbow and knee pads. This allows falling while minimising the damage. I found that this was more readily accepted in States than in Britain. I mentioned Jimmy Pollard previously, author of 'Hurry up and wait!'... (see references). Once he said to me, 'Do you want to know the difference between priorities in nursing in Britain and America? In Britain, the biggest word is dignity. In America the biggest word is freedom'. He meant that while both concepts were important in both countries, he had encountered a difference in emphasis. To be honest, I agree.

I saw people with quite advanced HD going out alone to shop and bank, kitted up like a cyclist or skate-boarder for safety. I saw a man fall over, get up and carry on in the street with no harm done. The risk was all assessed by a team, involving the client, and was written in the nursing plan. The benefits were shown to outweigh the potential for harm. I never saw this in Britain. But such a well considered plan would meet the requirements of our Health and safety legislation (Health and Safety at Work Act 1974), the Nursing and Midwifery Council Code of Conduct (NMC2000), and the Care Standards Act (2000). In the UK, the Mental Capacity Act (2005) and in other countries, similar legislation should be taken into account if there is concern that the person taking the risk might not have sufficient capacity to understand what the risk is, and what the consequences could be. This Act is considered below.

Members of staff need to allow people in their care to make their decisions, provided they have the capacity to do so. And we should be prepared to support decisions even if they are not decisions we would consider appropriate. On the other hand, we have a duty of care, and must ensure we act in the person's best interests especially when the person does not have capacity to make an informed decision, weighing potential risks against benefits. But this is a difficult balance to achieve. Planning the appropriate level of care needs to be a team effort involving the person, and where appropriate, an advocate should be identified. There's a bigger worry in my own country the UK, I think, about public perceptions than in the USA. Where I am I believe it is more likely that people in the street would be very upset that a client from a nursing home was in the street all by himself and obviously at the risk of falling, even if padded up for a fall. Skateboarders fall and are padded up to reduce the risk and still retain their dignity. So why not the person described above? My sweeping generalisation maybe wrong. It's my impression though after visiting many such nursing homes in both countries.

In the UK, as mentioned, the Mental Capacity Act (2005) was introduced to help in difficult situations such as these, and it is important to know five important principles of this legislation. They are:

1. Every adult has the right to make choices and decisions and should be presumed to have capacity unless it is proved otherwise.

2. People should be supported to make their own decisions as far as possible, before anyone assumes that they do not have the capacity.

3. There is a right to make what might be seen as unwise or eccentric decisions

4. Anything done on behalf of a person who lacks capacity must be in their best interests.

5. Anything done on behalf of a person lacking capacity must be the least restrictive approach, with regard to their basic rights and freedoms.

This Act and the responsibility to exercise a duty of care should inform any discussion about how to respond to risks taken by people who may lack capacity.

So, the right level of expertise must be consulted. There must be a careful plan, documented, monitored and evaluated, and there should be agreement between the experts, staff, the client, and where applicable, family or an advocate.

Other interventions to reduce the impact of harm from falls include rounding off the edges of furniture. One home had patched up a triangle shaped cut on a client's forehead several times, before someone realised the shape matched the edge of a bed side cabinet! The home's joiner shaved and sanded the corner and it never happened again. One poor lady fell while opening a door. Her hand was stuck in the handle lever and she hurt her wrist badly. The door handles were changed from levers to round knobs all over the home.

One home manager had got staff to walk around the home acting as if unsteady due to being 'drunk'. He noted the objects on which the staff most frequently bumped into, (bumped gently they were being careful really). He moved them, changed them, or got rid of them. He had a rubber padding fixed to small sections of the wall or corners that tended to get in the way. He didn't have any whole wall padded, just the little section that was likely to cause damage. I adapted his idea with a staff group; we felt that acting as though drunk might be perceived as though it was intended to denigrate the individuals, which of course it wasn't. We decided to act as though the room was a train carriage, travelling along a bumpy twisty route, and pretend we were trying to carry a tray of coffees. The result was the same, a lot of fun with furniture never previously regarded as obstacles being more critically considered.

No-one was trying, in either case, to compare people with a movement disorder with people who are drunk or on a train journey. But it was a way of looking at the potential problems associated with fixtures and fittings from a new perspective, allowing us to consider hazards previously unnoticed.

Some facilities are purpose-built. You lucky people! You can order everything made rounded or soft where needed. But the rest of us have to improvise. Some people prefer this situation, as some of these old properties have so much character.

Believe me, potential falls are well worth consideration,

before they start to happen. An efficient nurse will see the potential problem before it becomes an actual problem, and will build a nursing plan accordingly. Don't allow yourself if possible, to be surprised by something that was predictable. I once nursed a gentleman with severe chorea who had a fractured collar bone. Medication that reduced his movement made his life intolerable because along with the involuntary movement, he lost his voluntary control as well. So he volunteered to bear with the pain. We used a TENS machine (Transcutaneous Electrical nerve Stimulation) and other complementary methods, but the pain was severe. The experience has kept me on my guard since.

Fire Hazards

Elsie was sixty five and had been diagnosed with HD for eight years. She was now unable to walk, and her speech was badly affected so that only those who knew her well could understand her. She lived in a small nursing home for elderly people. Although the category 'elderly' kicks in at sixty four, those who knew her, knew that she felt out of place. She loved to laugh with the young carers, and didn't find much in common with the other older people. She'd lost her family. Don't get me wrong. They still visited and cared for and loved her very much. But she wasn't living among them anymore. They couldn't cope. That was probably the greatest of her many losses. But one thing she enjoyed was a cigarette. She was determined not to lose that one luxury in life. She had encountered some care professionals with other ideas.

Elsie's cigarettes had featured in some challenging situations over the last few years, and partly explained why she was now in a small home for elderly people rather than a large purpose built facility where her Social Worker had arranged her first unsuccessful placement. There was a smoking area set apart from other residents. Elsie had her cigarette in the right area, but when she'd finish, instead of putting the stub into the ashtray, she walked along the corridor and found a waste bin. At home, she had a metal waste bin and that's where she had always put cigarette ends. This bin was plastic and half full of paper. There was quite a large fire, but thankfully due to the prompt actions of the staff no one was hurt.

The home decided that Elsie posed too great a risk to the other residents, and the Social Worker was faced with finding an alternative. Every home she visited, on learning about a history of being moved on because of a fire risk, declined Elsie except the current home, where an increased fee was agreed to provide for sufficient staff to enable continual individual monitoring.

The trouble is, as this home found, no matter how many staff members you put on, you cannot be sure that someone like Elsie will be watched constantly. There are problems with ensuring whether Elsie has privacy and dignity. If the staff members keep her under close observation every moment, this can be upsetting for the staff members who feel that they are being made to act oppressively. Thankfully, by nature, the staff tend to recoil from engaging in activity that can be perceived as harassment or intrusive. Therefore, the monitoring needs to be discrete most of the time when checking and ensuring that there is no danger. Suddenly, when all backs are turned, the alarms go off, and Elsie is found hiding a lighted cigarette in a drawer full of bedding, because she senses someone will be annoyed if she's seen smoking outside the allocated area. Arguably in this instance, it might be less dangerous to permit smoking around the home.

They had a few close encounters like that, but the only time anyone was hurt was Elsie herself. It was when the person monitoring her lit a cigarette for her in the appropriate setting!

She had just had her hair done. As the staff member put the lighter to her cigarette, and tried to follow her jerking movement, she twisted her head, and suddenly her hair was alight. The quick thinking staff member threw a towel into the sink, and then threw it, soaked, over her head. This is not exactly as we are taught in the fire safety books and courses (please check). But it worked! Elsie had no eyebrows for a while, and a couple of small blisters appeared on her forehead, but nothing serious happened. Of course, the potential is very serious. Elsie's clothes were covered in ash burns from near misses.

The home was taking a chance and might not be forgiven if other residents were seriously harmed. Then one of the staff learned about a 'smoky Joe'. This is a contraption, which facilitates safer smoking for someone with chorea. A heavy ashtray sits on the table beside the client. The cigarette is placed into a hole on the inside wall of the ashtray. A tube runs from the outer wall, to a mouthpiece. The client smokes by holding the mouthpiece. The tube is flexible and allows for choreic movement. Any ash from the cigarette only drops into the ashtray.

Elsie didn't think much of the smoky Joe. But in a discussion, she understood that the alternatives were move to another home give up smoking or use the smoky Joe. A few times initially, Elsie broke the rules, by taking her cigarette out from the smoky Joe. The staff remained calm. They didn't get into an argument or recite ultimatums. They just offered to help her to put it back, 'before anyone sees', and she seemed to go along with it. As we saw before, one helpful effect of HD is that once something becomes routine, it tends to stick. This is true also of many people with other neurological conditions. Soon Elsie acted as though the only way to have a cigarette was via the smoky Joe.

This is a tricky subject, I know, with laws about preventing people smoking in public places including nursing homes and hospitals increasingly restricting the smoking habits.

The Principles

I have only, so far, highlighted the issues of falls and fire regarding safety. But of course, maintaining a safe environment is a massive topic. There are so many other dangers, some general, and some particularly significant in the context of advanced neurological disorders. But even though only two issues have been highlighted and not in any depth, hopefully it is possible to glean from them, the principles related to maintaining a safe environment.

How should nurses react if they don't agree with the concerns of the registration inspector? One resident continuously pulled the nurse call alarm. She didn't want to see the nurse when she got there. It was a persevering fixation with the bell, and the nurse coming in to ask how she was seemed to increase the client's agitation. The nurses decided to disconnect the bell, and made an alternative arrangement for regularly checking the client to see whether she was okay and had anything she wished for or needed. The client calmed down. The home inspector pointed out that this was not legal in that country. Every client must have access to a working call bell. It was re-connected and the difficulties re-commenced. A well-written risk assessment, demonstrating that all aspects have been considered may have helped the inspector and the nurse to agree about the best way forward.

Communication

Perhaps the reason that the central nervous system, the whole nervous system in fact seems so core to our being is that it is the system that so obviously communicates. All the systems communicate in some way, but in the nervous system this is so apparent. Signals or impulses travel from a cell body, stimulated by other cells down the axon, across the synapse to yet other cells, and in turn to muscles and to all areas of the body.

But beyond that the nervous system is our instrument for communication between ourselves and the world out there and all other people we have direct or remote contact with. And in the care of people who have impairment in this system, the effort to communicate effectively with them, two-way, is essential.

I have a rather sad story that I feel reflects the importance of good communication, which must include, naturally, listening to patients.

Mrs. Mercer was 63 and was in the hospital for assessment following a fall. She had Parkinson's disease. Her voice was very quiet due to the effort it took to use the muscles to force the air through her vocal cords. What she had to say was always intellectually sharp, often witty and interesting. Her daughter Jane visited her frequently. They had a chat and a few laughs, and then Mrs. Mercer explained that she needed to go to the toilet. Jane tried to flag down a couple of nurses as they went past, but they didn't seem to notice.

So Jane assisted her aunt, and soon they were back in the visiting area, with Mrs. Mercer in her wheelchair. 'Mum, what's happening with your assessment, and when will you be discharged?' Jane asked. Mrs. Mercer had no idea, and Jane went off to find out. A nurse explained that generally Mrs. Mercer seemed okay, but she was a bit confused, disorientated and agitated. The doctor was going to come in the morning and he would be asked to prescribe some medication for this.

Jane was astounded. 'My mother, confused...what makes you say that?' The nurse explained that, although they keep reminding Mrs. Mercer to stay sitting when they go past, she insists on standing up, and if she does she's likely to fall. Jane suggested that if she did stand up, Mrs. Mercer was more likely to fall after taking the medication. And she asked, 'Why do you think she's standing up?' The nurse replied, 'She's disorientated and confused. She forgets we've just told her to sit down'. But Jane explained, 'No, My mother asks you for the toilet, and you don't come to help her. So she has no choice but to try and stand and get there herself. I've just seen her try to ask you, and you and your colleague walked past. And Mum tells me she has this problem every time.'

'But we've told her', the nurse explained, 'She's wearing an incontinence pad; she doesn't have to go anywhere.' With that, Jane was furious. 'My mother is not about to sit in a lounge and urinate. A lot has gone wrong for her, but she hasn't given up on maintaining some dignity'.

There are a lot of issues in there—health and safety issues. There should be a good risk assessment. There should also be a specific falls risk assessment and these should be negotiated with the patient. There's the issue of neglect and misuse of aids to help with incontinence. Mrs. Mercer was not incontinent. She could get to the toilet with some help. But underpinning all of that was the problem of a lack of communication; failing to take time to listen and to demonstrate a willingness to address needs as perceived by the patient.

Now, the health professionals have taken some criticism in this book. But mostly the interventions reported here are excellent and very helpful. It's right to also mention things we don't do so well. That's how we learn and improve. Most care I witness is above and beyond the call of duty. Thanks to all good caring and dedicated health professionals.

Eating and Drinking

Sometimes, in a nursing plan, instead of a section on eating and drinking, I have noticed headings such as 'nutrition', or 'diet'. I feel that the dietician maybe justified in considering this activity in those terms. But from a nursing perspective, I rather think it misses the point. Awareness of dietary needs, to ensure adequate nutrition is certainly important and is an important part of what we need to consider. But eating and drinking is a much broader activity than that. When you think about why you eat and drink, you can come up with a range of reasons depending on the context.

Did you stop for breakfast before you went to work? Why was that?

Were you invited to a restaurant by a colleague? Why was that?

Did you bring a packed lunch? Were you at the Christmas dinner?

They all raise different issues about why you may eat and drink on a particular occasion.

If we build a nursing plan around nutrition and diet, we are in danger of limiting the scope of our care to exclude many of these important issues. That may explain why I found that a man who had been fitted with a 'gastrostomy' tube, never saw the dining room in his nursing home again. This is a tube connected to a bag of liquid containing the necessary nutrients for life. The tube is inserted into the stomach via a surgically made opening in the abdomen. A machine ensures the tube supplies the nutrition at the prescribed rate. This can reduce some of the danger of choking, and of starving due to difficulties in swallowing, that can arise in the later stages of degenerative neurological conditions. The tube is often referred to as a PEG tube (percutaneous endoscopic gastrostomy) and will be discussed a little more later.

Whatever way the heading is worded, ('Diet' 'Nutrition', or as I find preferable 'Eating and Drinking') this tends to be a section in any nursing plan where problems are identified. But perhaps the nature of the problem is not always as clearly thought through as it could be, to help with planning what can be done about it. Some of the problems I often see recorded include that he or she:

1. Spits out food

2. Throws the plate off the table

3. Has a tendency to choke

4. Dribbles

5. Dislikes most foods

6. Is unable to eat / drink / swallow

I have also occasionally seen opinions recorded, suggesting that he or she is demonstrating that they no longer want to live by refusing food. When I have seen this, it has been in the context of someone who is unable to speak sufficiently well to confirm or refute this to staff, other professionals or relatives. In particular, I have noticed these remarks made in the context of decision-making regarding whether or not a PEG tube should be considered.

I'm sure in the instances when I have come across these statements in nursing plans for clients with neurological disease that they are truthful and accurate. It's just that they don't really give enough of an explanation to be able to work with. This can leave the staff member who tries to work with the plan, feeling defeated. What on earth can you do about someone who spits out food? Don't sit too close? Put a plastic sheet over the table cloth and carpet? Don't give her any food? None of it seems constructive, and there doesn't seem to be the opportunity to enjoy the rewards that should come with individualised nursing. But that's only because of the way the problems have been presented as facts about the person. They could be presented more as a challenge to the staff, or to the carer at home as the case maybe.

For example, in the case of trying to help a person with an advanced degenerative neurological condition to eat, who seems at times to be spitting out the food, it can be helpful to sit coolly at a time when you're not feeling too upset by it, and try to establish whether there might be a pattern to this. You could consider whether this tends to occur more often with certain types of food. It maybe that he or she doesn't like these foods anymore, even if they were once their favourites. Perhaps, they have become difficult to manage to chew or because of changes in taste perception, or ability to handle the texture, they just seem to be unpalatable. You could check whether there maybe a relationship between the 'spitting out' and the amount loaded onto a fork or spoon or the time between taking mouthfuls. This would be easy to change and experiment with. Sorry if this seems a bit patronising. I know you could feel a bit understandably annoyed reading this if you're thinking, of course I've tried all of this, it's obvious. Please bear with me if that's the case, as it can often happen to people that the role of caring can become so draining with tasks like helping someone to eat so repetitive, that it's really easy to overlook the obvious. The changes happen so gradually, that it's not easy to stand back from the situation and take a fresh look at it. A different observation might be that the 'spitting out' might be happening as an automatic (and therefore consistent) response to the introduction of food to the mouth.

Having made the observations, it is best to seek a speech therapy assessment to establish the level of ability to swallow food, and get advice regarding the food texture and tips on assisting to eat and drink. The speech and language therapist will be likely to appreciate the help to clarify what the problem is and how best to work with you to alleviate it, rather than just start with a comparatively vague description of spitting out food.

Perhaps the 'spitting' problem will be resolved by reverting to the person being more independent, and allowing for some spillage, as long as she or he is able to manage to eat satisfactorily. This can help.

Maybe on the other hand, it will turn out that the person you are caring for is so hungry that he or she is trying to get food down quicker than is manageable. But it could instead turn out to be due to problems with muscular coordination with the tongue protruding when the individual intends to draw it down and back. In this case, food would be pushed out involuntarily. Maybe, the spoon is being loaded again too soon after swallowing, or the whole process, though seeming slow to the carer is too rushed from the perception of the individual concerned. Perhaps the staff are too fast with feeding, or are loading up the spoon too much. There must be many other avenues to explore. When an answer is found, there can be a real sense of satisfaction all round. The relief can be as great for the carer as for the person being cared for.

An important thing is not to start worrying that a change in how you're helping might mean that somehow, you've been 'doing it wrong'. I think that natural fear is what can stop a lot of people considering adjustments that might be needed. You haven't been 'doing it wrong', but the nature of the condition, whatever the degenerative neurological diagnosis, is that ability, perception, taste and so on change, and what was a fine way to work may need to be modified, often by trial and error.

Many people who have movement disorders that involve continued involuntary movements such as chorea in Huntington's disease complain that their hunger is never satisfied. One fellow I knew, Roger, who was six feet tall and slim, started each day with seven wheat biscuits covered in sugar, calorie supplement powder, and covered in cream rather than milk. One famous company who make this breakfast cereal based an advertising campaign on the assertion that it was not possible to eat three! Roger would down the lot, then have bacon, eggs and baked beans. He would often put the cutlery down and use his hands to try and get it into his mouth faster. One day when he choked on a sausage, a carer saved his life. She alternated between giving five backslaps and 'abdominal thrusts' as she had learned in the First Aid classes.

I'm sure this desperation to eat so much and cram it in so fast was largely because of the long wait from evening supper (often early because some residents liked to go to bed early). At that time, there was a mentality that all the residents should eat at the same time. More frequently available, not so large meals would have saved the situation from arising I feel. Roger was very down at times about his condition, and had even expressed a wish to die. But he never forgot the carer's swift and calm action, and he was so grateful to her. Choking, I'm sure you are aware is an extremely frightening experience.

There is a danger however, that because carers are worried about causing choking, they may sometimes be afraid to assist a person with advanced neurological disease to eat and drink sufficiently. It is often said that people with advanced Huntington's disease for example, need 5000 calories daily to maintain their body weight, which is considered to be related to the ability to postpone disability, or incapacity. If Roger's meals were delayed, he could become very upset and could hit too. Sometimes, despite his hunger, he would throw the meal away when it arrived through sheer frustration. The staff team were smart enough to realise not to bother about trying to manage the behaviour. They just made sure the delay didn't happen very often.

In most centres now, I'm happy to say, there has been a move away from sticking only to rigid meal times. Many people with advanced neurological conditions manage hunger better if they have frequent, smaller, high calorie snacks, rather than three or four big meals daily. And it can be good for some individuals to make sure that night time snacks, hot or cold are always at the ready. These are good developments, and as indicated by Roger's case, can help to avoid situations where people are panicking to cram food into their mouths faster than they can manage swallowing. Some facilities that run very good activity programmes often plan the snacks into an agenda of short activity sessions. One day at a nursing home, I attended the various sessions on offer along with the residents. I had coffee and shortbread in a prayer meeting; pancakes and maple syrup at an art class; choc-ice at a discussion group; trifle in a music and movement session, and then stopped for lunch. The afternoon programme was equally satisfying! I didn't tell my wife and still ate dinner at home!

There are many benefits to stalling off weight loss which occurs in many people who are declining neurologically. Regarding HD particularly, people tend to report feeling fitter, and medication is thought to be more effective as a result (Pollard, 2003). We have been considering people who spend energy all day on involuntary movement and consequently are hungry and seem to eat excessively, but of course with other neurological problems, sluggishness and apathy can result in no real interest in food at all. Certainly these individuals tend to be put off by the sight of a large plate of food. So once again, frequent, light, appetising nutritious snacks are likely to be more appreciated.

When Roger's HD was more advanced, he needed more assistance to eat and drink. He also needed a different, specialised chair to enable him to adopt a posture conducive to easier swallowing. He was a guy who, like most of us would probably be, was keen to hang on to his independence. He didn't like being 'fed' and wanted to use the same kind of chair as everyone else in the dining room.

Fortunately, those staff members who had worked there for some time and had built up a rapport with Roger were able to anticipate this set of circumstances before they arose. They didn't suddenly change everything in the course of a week or month. They gradually got Roger accustomed to the chair (on wheels) away from the dining area. They picked an opportunity when he was tired one time, and asked if he'd like to go just for once on the chair, never suggesting he needed to get used to it. It was some time before that happened again. But gradually it began to occur fairly frequently. The time came when he had got so used to having meals in his new chair that he refused to sit in the ordinary dining chair. There was much more chance of concordance when it became his choice rather than an idea insisted on by the nursing team. Notice I didn't use the word often heard, 'compliance'. You won't win with the people I've met who have any neurological condition affecting the abilities reliant on the brain's frontal lobe to control impulses and see other people's point of view, if you go down that track! Work to achieve 'concordance' rather than 'compliance'.

You will recognise if and when swallowing becomes problematic by observing effort in trying to chew, constant throat clearing, and food being still in the mouth after several swallows. The voice might have a 'wet gurgling' sound. Weight loss may start to become obvious with clothes becoming looser and often after a meal, the person you are caring for is exhausted through the sheer effort of having to work to coordinate the necessary muscular movement and avoid asphyxiation. This situation indicates a need for an increased level of intervention. Call in the experts earlier rather than later.

The speech therapist will help you to assess the swallowing and will make recommendations about the food and drink texture, and the types of food that can be managed. She or he will also help to find the optimum positioning to make eating and swallowing easier. The Dietician will help assess dietary need and nutritional status, and will help to suggest menus that meet the needs, taking account of the speech therapists assessment of capability and limitations. The Physiotherapist will help to increase independence by maximising the range of movement and will advise on positioning. Chest physiotherapy (that's our UK word for 'Physical Therapy') maybe provided to reduce the likelihood of pneumonia to which the client is vulnerable because of the tendency to aspirate. The Occupational Therapist will help to maximise independence also by helping to organise the environment, and provide utensils and other equipment, to make the most use of what range of movement and level of stability exists.

As emphasised previously, the interdisciplinary team members are so valuable, you need to involve them early and not wait until there is a nutritional or hydration crisis.

One very obliging speech therapist, with the client's consent obviously, arranged a video fluoroscopy for teaching purposes. A video fluoroscopy allows us to view what actually happens inside the mouth when the person is trying to swallow. It is usually done when the speech therapist finds it necessary to help with making an assessment. But on this occasion, we found it useful as part of our education. We could see how long it took to move the food around with the tongue until it became a formed bolus ready to swallow. Then we saw that as it was about to move to the back of the throat, the lips would lose their hold and the food would be pushed out instead of backwards to enable swallowing. We saw that un-thickened drinks were dangerously running past the epiglottis down towards the lungs.

Nurses and other care staff who watched this said that although they had been told about these things, they were now clearer about the problems, and would find it easier to have the patience to allow time to clear the mouth before introducing more food or drink. The speech therapist felt that trying for 20-25 minutes was hard enough work, and that other methods of obtaining adequate nutrition should be sought if they couldn't get it in that time.

The time is likely to come for a lot of people with a degenerative neurological disorder when pureed food is recommended. Depending on how this is served, it can put people off eating altogether. The company which make the thickener for drinks for the homes I have worked in, in England and Scotland make moulds, and run free teaching sessions to show how the thickener can be mixed with the pureed food so that it is cooked and served in its recognisable form. Pureed chicken in the shape of a leg, peas looking like a little pile of peas, and so on, all in the desired consistency. Do speak to a company representative. I have found that they tend to be keen to offer ideas of how to achieve this even if a company don't supply the moulds or teaching. I first saw these moulds in use in United States. So they are no doubt available almost globally. So, please try to avoid serving a plate full of unrecognisable mush!

This discussion does lead onto the issue of feeding tubes or 'PEG' tubes, or as has become more common in some areas, Jejunostomy tubes that are inserted into the small intestine, that is, beyond the stomach. Decisions about whether this is a good idea in individual cases are difficult and are discussed in the section further on, called 'Big Decisions'.

Whatever the decision might be, what must be clear are the reasons for considering the tube in the first place. This is where the therapists can help nurses to check that we are clear that there is a sufficient nutritional or hydration crisis to justify the intervention, or that the risk of aspiration or choking is serious. Perhaps the individual has ceased to enjoy eating and drinking because of the fear of choking. Also, the therapists can help to confirm that all the possible less intrusive methods such as improved positioning, relaxing environment, ideal consistency of food and drink etc, have been tried.

A couple of things to remember about tube feeding is that it doesn't always have to replace eating and drinking orally. It can provide the extra needed, when the effort of managing a meal becomes too great. Even when total parenteral feeding is necessary, it is usually possible to introduce a range of tastes to the mouth. There is no reason not to enjoy the social aspect of eating. Many will enjoy coming to lunch, and join in the banter, while having a small taster. Guidance from the therapists is crucial. If it is upsetting to see people eat orally when unable to do the same, staff need to compensate by having a time when the social aspect is compensated for in some other way, perhaps by sitting with the client when offering mouth care, and chatting, in an area set aside.

Do not automatically exclude a tube-fed resident at your home, from a trip out to a restaurant. Choice and individuality are key.

Continence Management

Until the very advanced stages, most people with neurological conditions that I have met, seem to be able to maintain continence both of urine and faeces, provided environmental factors are considered and addressed. Problems can arise though in conditions that interfere with neurological signals between the brain and the bladder, or sphincters (circular muscle bands that surround openings) controlling the flow of urine or in the rectum and anus, the control of faeces. Multiple sclerosis is one example of a condition in which for some people, the once easily controlled activities of passing urine or faces can develop into a problem to manage. Conditions that cause people to lose cognition and insight can lead to incontinence even if the relevant muscles of the urinary and digestive systems and the neural pathways connecting them to the brain are intact.

This is because in those conditions attention can become increasingly focussed on immediate needs, and so they may not foresee that 'now' might be a good time to go, because 'later' might be awkward for some reason. Perhaps a number of people in a nursing home for example, are going to need to take a bath consecutively, or the staff will be busy preparing lunch. Failure to rationalise in this way means that by the time the impulse is strong enough to prompt the person to act, it will definitely be the time to go!

Our job is to make sure that's going to be possible. Many care homes now have en-suite facilities. In the day around the home, we need to consider the potential problem when planning the day, and organising seating arrangements etc. I met a lady whose nursing plan indicated that she had urinary urgency, causing occasional incontinence. The staff members were quite frustrated with her because she would not accept wearing a pad. They tried all sizes and shapes but she kept pulling at them till they fell to pieces, leaving fluff all over the home. In another facility, some notes in a nursing plan suggested that a man in his mid forties with impaired frontal lobe functioning was exhibiting bizarre ritualistic behavior involving the smearing of excrement on the walls.

These people were not bizarre. The damage to neural pathways involving the frontal part of the brain causes difficulty in planning ahead, considering alternatives, and suppressing impulses. These are all skills necessary to enable someone to wait for a convenient time or get in earlier or to put up with wearing uncomfortable and restrictive incontinence pads. They were just trying to get those things off. The gentleman in doing so, was finding that his hands were covered in faeces. In desperation he rubbed his hands anywhere to get rid of the mess. The walls just happened to be a surface within easy reach. There turned out to be no strange ritual, but rather, a logical attempt to resolve the problem.

See how easily a misunderstanding like that on the part of professionals, who might have failed to discover the reason for the 'behaviour' could have resulted in the person being prescribed anti-psychotic medication. Apart from probably making a person with no psychotic symptoms endure side effects and aggravating problems with confusion and cognition, we might well end up causing constipation. Yes, when we're not careful our treatments can be worse than the conditions we have set out to treat.

If you keep reminding yourself that cognitive decline is not a mental illness, it is the result of a degenerative neurological disease, it can help you to work out answers to what may seem like bizarre behaviour. This means that normally when you get to the bottom of it, there will be a rational explanation. I say 'normally' because clearly it isn't the case every time. Psychiatric disorder can occur with florid psychotic episodes. But in my experience, when you see a reliable pattern in the activity, you should expect to be able to make sense of it, and then find the answer.

Other than this, the normal nursing response to incontinence is appropriate whenever it occurs as a problem. That is, find out the cause and resolve it. Is there a urinary tract infection? A neurogenic bladder? Retention? Is sleepiness or lethargy stopping the individual from getting there on time? These problems maybe caused or aggravated by antidepressants or any other medication acting on the central nervous system.

Of course, constipation may occur also, whether or not we cause it by giving inappropriate medication as discussed above. Again, find the cause, suspect medication, poor diet, insufficient fluids, lack of fruit intake and exercise. With unresolved problems related to eliminating, bring in the continence adviser. This should not be seen as a problem to be expected and tolerated. In the very last stages of neurological deteriorating disease of course, incontinence is likely, just as with anyone who is so ill and confined to bed. The normal high standard of nursing care for the dying patient with attention to comfort and hygiene is appropriate.

For mobile people with cognitive and movement problems, falls and other accidents are a risk when going to the toilet. Hurrying to get there on time, turning on the spot to sit, while partly undressing is tricky enough for anyone to negotiate; but it will particularly be difficult for a person who has a movement disorder, poor balance, cannot concentrate on more than one thing at a time, and whose visuo-spatial awareness is impaired. Visuo-spatial awareness is that sense that gives us a steady map of the room and our position in it, even though we can't see much of it as we turn and move around. This is that sense which apart from causing other navigating difficulties, can lead to someone being assisted to turn and to sit down, becoming frightened and locked into a stiff body posture, resisting the effort to get them onto the chair or toilet seat. It takes patience and a reassuring assistant to help the individual to gain the confidence needed to become supple in the middle, and sit back onto the toilet.

There is of course a gender issue here. Turning to sit can be a problem, and men, trying to stand and pass urine may have particular difficulty. There is often a mess. If he doesn't want to get used to sitting, don't persist. Eventually, he probably will. Nursing homes need to ensure there is a spacious bathroom with bright lighting and easy to clean surrounding, but not slippery floors. This maybe less easy at home of course, and can be a reason for nursing (or residential care home) admission. Make sure there are no sharp or pointed edges and corners on baths, sinks and other fittings. Don't fuss or react to the spillage. It's no one's fault. These days in a bathroom with modern facilities, it should be easy to clean up without any hygiene risk to yourself. A home that is not equipped may not be a suitable placement. However, when I ran one particular small home for young people with neurological disorders, I received funding to make necessary changes, once I'd clearly set out the case. It was less expensive for the health services to support that than find somewhere else, and less disruptive to the life of a resident who was enjoying a good quality of life at the home.

Fittings in the bathroom need to be pretty robust. A person with chorea can easily break a few cheap toilet seats in a week. Get the disability equipment company representatives to come out and compete with demonstrations. Tell them in advance what the problems are and get them thinking. I've seen some marvellous innovations, individually made by some companies to get round tricky problems. Then again, in one establishment I visited, they believed in buying cheap plastic toilet seats. This meant that when a person with chorea moved around, the seat gave way a little and moved with the person, while the fitment remained still. This prevented the bolts lifting out of the floor. They replaced the seats frequently, checking carefully for signs of an impending split that might cause an injury. It must be possible to manufacture a tough seat with a bit of leeway?

Washing and Dressing

Let's briefly contemplate the great questions that I find crop up often, and can be divisive among some nursing teams:

1. Is a shower better than a bath?

2. Which is a better time to take a shower—morning, afternoon or evening?

3. How often should someone have a bath or a shower?

4. Is it acceptable to sit in the day room or eat in the dining room with the other guests in a dressing gown, pyjamas, or a nightgown?

You may as well argue about, 'How long is a piece of string?' Of course, from a biological perspective, a shower maybe cleaner, because in a bath you are surrounded by the dirt washed off the body. You could always rinse off, I guess. Baths use more water. But to some, they are the ultimate relaxation. It is usually easier physically to get someone into a shower. A bath, and particularly some specially adapted baths could be argued to be safer for someone with movement disorder and poor balance. When limbs fly out due to chorea, there maybe more chance of being hit when trying to assist with a shower, than if the individual was in a bath. And what is wrong with an all-over wash on a chair by the sink, or a bed bath anyway, for someone who is at the risk of falling and injuring himself?

Many more arguments for and against baths and showers are possible and valid, and the same could be said with regard to the other questions. What is important is to work with the resident to reach the most agreeable decision. Staff should remain flexible, as the client may well have lost the ability to be as adaptable. The rights of one resident in a home to make a choice need to be balanced against the rights of the others to be safe, and not to be offended; and vice versa.

In one home, the staff team were reprimanded by a visiting inspector because a resident walked through the living room in her dressing gown at 4pm. The inspector felt that staff members were getting people ready for bed early so that they could have an easier shift after the evening meal had been served and cleared away. The team were offended, and pointed out in a well-written nursing plan that it was identified as the lady's choice to have a shower at that time and spend the evening in a dressing gown. Because of chorea, the lady felt much more comfortable in loose clothing, and liked to have a day in a track suit, followed by an evening in a dressing gown. The inspector was won over with the notion that the clothing was a matter of the resident's choice, mainly because the process in establishing the choice was carefully documented.

However, she did not accept the argument that taking a shower at 4pm, in this case, was an independent choice. She had asked the lady what time she preferred to take a shower, and, indeed, the lady answered 4pm. The inspector concluded that the answer was a result of institutionalisation, and could not be considered a choice. She knew enough to realise that people with declining cognition often tend to get into a routine that they feel safer with and don't like to break, and she advised against trying to change a pattern. But she remained suspicious about how the routine got there in the first place and for whose benefit.

Who would have inspectors? Of course, she was concerned to get the staff beyond the idea of thinking that free choice is just a matter of getting someone to come out with a particular response. But there was a real danger here, of deflating a staff team who had done very well to get a routine going that worked and kept everybody happy. She maybe didn't appreciate just how difficult that can be, and how soul-destroying it can be to hear someone call the effort into question. But this particular team had learned a great combined skill. They were not demoralised by other's opinions especially by an outsider's view. In fact, they welcomed it as an opportunity to check the reasons behind their nursing planning. I sat with them after this inspection visit, and I expected them to get defensive, but that didn't happen. After carefully considering the possibility that institutionalisation was a potential problem, limiting the choices the residents were able to make, they concluded it was a valid point to be aware of, but stayed with the plan for the lady concerned. Good for them!

How much individuals can do for themselves is often the subject of difficult decisions. A careful individualised assessment is necessary involving the Physiotherapist to see what range of movement we should be encouraging, and the Occupational Therapist to see whether we have adapted the environment sufficiently to maximise independence, and are using the appropriate equipment where necessary. It is definitely true that a spacious bathroom / washroom / W.C. is imperative. There must be no sharp corners or edges or pointed protrusions. The floor must be easy to clean but not slippery. There must be plenty of good light and few shadows.

I do mention nursing and care homes often, not because I'm not thinking of you all who are caring at home, but because the issues that arise in those facilities often make good examples to think about in all sorts of caring situations including at home.

Well in this instance, if you do not think you have bathing and washing and toilet facilities that come up to the ideal standard, press your social worker to sort out the finance and the provision of better equipment and if necessary, the building of an extension. I am sure he or she will be happier to arrange that than to find a placement in a care home just because your bathroom is not practical for the role you are expected to undertake.

There is a great deal of clothing that can make it easier for some individuals to dress themselves with little intervention. As the lady described above found it is generally better to go for fairly loose clothing, and many prefer track suits or baggy trousers and T shirts. For people who need changing often, it is possible to get shirts or trousers with a front that comes off, so that there is no need to be pulling arms out of sleeves just because of a soup spill at lunch, or making a person who can hardly stand get out of a chair just because of a wet lap.

For many, Velcro and zips add a lot of independence compared to buttons. Slip on shoes can save having someone to do up laces.

Where we do have to intervene, it's a good practice I feel, to let the person do the finishing touches. You may recall that earlier I mentioned that when helping someone to shave, if I think they can manage part of it, but won't be able to get under the nose, or lower lip or whatever, I ask if they mind me doing it first. Then the person takes over using a mirror. If I think it's still not quite neat, I'll remember for the next time, but I won't interfere. Well similarly, I would have to think carefully about whether it's worth telling someone who has independently dressed that buttons are misaligned, or a T-shirt is inside-out. If it's going to detract from dignity, then perhaps I'll sensitively and discretely find a chance to help put it right. But otherwise, if he's happy, that's the bottom line. He has the satisfaction of being in control of the final product. Self-esteem is worth more than straightening out a few rough edges.

Mouth care is so important. Electric toothbrushes are useful to some people with difficulty in fine motor control. It gets to the places where they wouldn't be able to give a good scrub manually. Regular, three to four monthly visits to the dentist are important, and are often neglected in some facilities for long term care in my experience. Dentures are only useful if they fit well. Many people find it easier to do without them for eating, but put them in afterwards for appearances. Like all of the above, it's a very individual thing.

Good skin care is essential. Impaired communicating may often mean that the person cannot indicate when clothing is rubbing on skin, or when there is itchiness or a rash. So we must keep checking. Are shoes too tight? Check for redness. In the advanced stages, weight loss leading to protruding bony prominences, and lengthy spells in a seat or in bed complicated by incontinence, will all lead to a high risk of pressure sore development. Regular turning, good hygiene practice and appropriate cushions and mattresses are essential along with constantly updated assessment.

Expressing Sexuality

We constantly express our sexuality, in so many areas of our lives and mostly we are unaware of doing so. Gender is much more than a fact of biology. We declare our masculinity or femininity in the clothing we wear, our hairstyle, in the friends we make and in the subjects we choose to discuss. Our posture, voice tone and facial expressions send out signals that tell those around us about our identity, of which our gender and orientation are an integral part. This is noticeable in every culture. The response we get in return for those signals helps us to reaffirm who we are to ourselves. It's good to feel comfortable with it.

The symptoms of neurological disorders can strike at every aspect of a person's sense of self and sexuality. Movement disorder, impaired speech and body language, incontinence, spilling food and making involuntary noises can all impact negatively on self esteem, as can the fact of living in a nursing home away from loved ones. We cannot get rid of the symptoms, but we can sometimes successfully reduce them. We can certainly break the negative feedback loop by sending back positive signals. We needn't do this by pretending, but by responding to the person, for who she or he is, and what he or she is trying to say, rather than to the impairment.

Hopefully, in this book so far, the importance of spending time with individuals, and attending to the aspects of care such as helping the client choose clothing, hair style, make up that enhances the person's individuality and dignity has been emphasised. The time spent and the amount of concern and interest shown by staff is as important as the detail concerning what styles are eventually decided upon.

Outings should be chosen according to one's personality. A lady who likes to perceive herself as very feminine may choose to see a romantic movie rather than go to the speedway. Not necessarily of course, it has to be about individual choice, but if being feminine in this case is an attribute under threat, it can become important to shore it up, with greater emphasis than might be necessary if there were sufficient compensating factors.

For example, if I'm out, I'd like a pint of beer. But if you bought me wine in a glass with a dainty stem, I'd be happy too. That's because I quite like wine, and I don't see why just because there's a past tradition about the difference between drinks for girls and for boys it should matter to me. We're all enlightened now about equality. But if my ability to express sexuality was impaired, I might take a different view. I might have to turn to some traditional props to ensure I sent out the signals I wanted to having lost the other ways of doing so. You may not agree with this. That's fine, I understand, and although I hold the view, I admit having misgivings about it. The point was included here not so much to convey a view, as to stimulate thought and debate.

You need to think about the consequences of lending someone a typically female or male umbrella on an outing. Perhaps, you or I would get away with it, and feel confident still about who we are. But in the absence of the compensating factors, will it demean the person? What about sitting on a big bus with an advert for a charity on the side? What about cartoon stickers on a wheelchair? It's only fun? Or can a lot of work to shore up dignity be undone pretty quickly? Again, I don't have answers. These are questions to pose, so that you can work towards considered responses appropriate to the individual. I do feel pretty sure that I wouldn't want to be seen waving from the window of a 'Sunshine' bus, or with stickers on my wheelchair if I were to use one. But, I know people who love all that.

I often hear people talk about inappropriate sexual behaviour and certainly I've encountered a number of difficult situations where the loss of inhibition due to cognitive deterioration has been problematic. But more often I feel, people seem to lose interest in sexual activity, perhaps in some cases because of exhaustion, lethargy and depression, low self esteem and the effects of medication.

Here is an account, told to a group of us (nurses) by the wife of a nursing home resident:

'When Dave lived at home we had slept apart for some time. He was constantly moving and the bed just wasn't big enough. Apart from that I think he knew that I just couldn't look at him in that way anymore. I felt so guilty, though I love him dearly, but I just couldn't. He made hideous facial grimaces, and the most awful grunting noises.

For a while he seemed to accept this. But I knew he was crying inside. So was I. Later on, he used to try and talk me around, but he had lost the ability to be subtle. Sometimes he would start grabbing me and fondling. Sometimes he hurt me. He didn't mean to be rough, but he was, and I couldn't help but push him away especially when he tried to kiss me. It was a nightmare. This made him angry. Sometimes he threw things around the room, slammed the door and stormed off to his bed.

At the nursing home I made friends with another woman of my age who shared a similar experience with me. It helped to talk about it. She told me that she actually has sex with her husband in his room. It took her a year thinking about it, because he was so frustrated and was sexually harassing the nurses. She said it was awful, but he calmed down, and didn't need to keep having medication for his behaviour, which made him drowsy and flattened his personality. But one day, a nurse had come into the room without knocking and reacted with shock. My friend said she felt dirty every time the staff looked at her after that.

I could never do what my friend did, but I admire her. There isn't any privacy, and I feel that the nurses would regard me as disgusting.'

I've seen homes where active sexual relationships between consenting residents is quietly encouraged and facilitated. There were also homes where it seemed to be actively prevented, although if asked, I feel the staff would deny this was the case. I have been interested in the way different staff deal with situations where clients strip off in public, often just to do with the feeling of restriction of clothing; or make suggestive comments and obscene jokes. It can cause a lot of friction when staff members disagree, with some joining in the jokes, saying that it's only fair to encourage a bit of fun, when people don't have many joys left, while others see it as demeaning.

I know of a nurse who lost his job after taking some residents to a prostitute. In fact, this led to the home's closure. A doctor once told me that he thought that if we were allowed to bring a prostitute into the home, he could cut out most of the medication he prescribes for 'aggressive behaviour'. 'It's really for frustration' he said.

I knew a young lady in her mid twenties who had HD. She was very attractive and took great care over her appearance. She had very many boyfriends, and sometimes went missing from her nursing home. The young lady often walked for miles, got lifts, and disappeared for days together. There were serious legal and ethical debates involving experts, concerning whether if she chose to go off on her own she should be able to, or whether the home had the right and the duty to provide greater protection. Psychiatrists had judged that she was competent to make choices and understood the risks. Staff at the home were deeply distressed about her vulnerability, and eventually declared that they could no longer look after her, as they were not allowed to lock doors, or insist on accompanying her against her will. **[Important: Please see the earlier comments on the Mental Capacity Act, 2005]**

I caught up with the same lady about five years later in another home many miles from the first. She was by now confined to bed, and was in a poor condition. I felt that she had a twinkle in her eye. She'd lived on the edge and the nurses who got to know her felt that there were no regrets.

However individuals choose to express sexuality, the staff at a nursing home should not sweep the matter under the carpet. There are clearly implications for providing access to good contraceptive advice. This is often forgotten.

If you're hoping I've got answers to these and many more questions and problems related to expressing sexuality, I'm afraid I'm going to let you down. All I can say is that wherever I have visited, the staff team tell me about all these kinds of issues. Yet, when I look at nursing plans, I don't often find evidence that the issues are out in the open. That would be a good starting point.

When people are frustrated, we can help to reduce this by hearing what they have to say, rather than ignoring it out of embarrassment, changing the subject, or making jokes about sexuality. Human contact in a manner that shows we care but cannot be construed as sexual is important, and is missing in the lives of many people in nursing homes. Aromatherapy and therapeutic massage can be good ways of giving human contact in a calming, professional way. A busy activity schedule that is meaningful will help. Most of all, we can help by trying our best to show empathy, love for fellow being, by taking time to listen and working to build self esteem.

Although I have not answered your problems, at least you should be sure you are not alone. Most of us have encountered similar situations, and hopefully there is some comfort in that. You must be clear that your job – whether you're paid to be a carer or a professional nurse, or are caring at home for a partner or other family member, neighbour or friend does not involve having to tolerate any kind of abuse. Just because a person cannot help it, it doesn't mean you'll have to put up with it.

That is why it is so important the issues are discussed as a group. The solution maybe difficult, but it must be resolved. Perhaps, your facility doesn't have the right environment, or doesn't have enough staff with appropriate training to deal with these situations. It is no failure if as a group, you have to decide that a resident would fare better elsewhere. No home can be suitable for every resident. For home carers, perhaps it is becoming unsustainable to carry on doing this in your own domestic environment. Painful though it might be, there's no failure in facing reality. You should discuss it with your social worker, or the specialist nurse, or the GP (family doctor). Leave them with no doubt if you can't go on.

Likewise, the people you are caring for are vulnerable to being abused, sexually or otherwise. People who cannot speak up for themselves are an obvious target for someone who wishes to do harm. Unfortunately, the reality is that some people who do intend to take advantage of someone's vulnerability will seek a job in a nursing or residential home, or perhaps as a visiting home carer. The nursing plan should identify this potential problem. Everyone should be aware.

A potential perpetrator should know that this is a group of staff or a family carer who will not sweep issues under the carpet; everything is out in the open. Bullies and abusers tend to steer clear of such an environment. If you do suspect that someone goes out of their way to bathe a certain person, or spends a long time dressing them or for no reason you can be sure of, you have an uneasy feeling, take your concerns to the management. Don't bottle it up. They should be trained to deal with it efficiently and discretely. The staff should know that this is how the team works. So anyone questioned who is doing no harm, should not feel offended, but pleased to know that we're busy making sure our clients are safe.

Sleeping

'At Last!' These are the words I have often found myself muttering quietly on a night duty, when I would see that one of our most restless clients had finally dropped off to sleep.

Generally, I find that people with advanced degenerative neurological conditions are exhausted most of the time. The constant movement, the burning up of calories for people with chorea, or the effort to make any effective movement in people with Parkinson's or Multiple Sclerosis; the enormous effort involved in keeping upright, balancing, eating and drinking while struggling to avoid choking, and giving all the lungs have to give to try and say something, is a years work done in a day. But despite the tiredness, exhaustion and weariness, it's often still more effort to try and get off to sleep.

It's not easy to sleep when you're uncomfortable but unable to move or in pain, as some people with conditions such as MS complain of at night; or still starving, despite having eaten for an army. It's not easy when you can't keep still and either keep banging limbs on the bed sides or fall out. And just as you manage to doze, there's a mighty crash and the person in the next room is apparently having the same trouble. So you get up to find the nurse. She or he is pretty weary too. You are told that you already had something to eat. You were tucked up only ten minutes ago, and the new sheets are wet already. You may have lost insight and some of the ability to view from another person's perspective. But you can just read body language and voice intonation well enough to realise that you're currently just a little less than welcome.

Despite the fact that there is a dedicated nurse who cares deeply about you, she or he is just another tired human being. Hopefully, he or she will conjure up the effort to help you settle again.

When the residents are all asleep (though it doesn't always happen of course) it's a good time for the nursing team to compliment themselves on the marvellous job that they are doing. Time to care for the carers. Very well done, you're special people. I've been so inspired working alongside people like yourselves. I wasn't that good at much of the hands on work to be honest. My bed-making was appalling. Thank God for quilts. They came in and saved me from constant criticism of my miss-aligned 'hospital corners'. I could never remember what I'd gone to the cupboard for and so on. So I was very dependent on the great teams working around me. And as compensation, at a time like this in the dead of night, with all quiet in the bedrooms, I made the warm drinks and toasts.

There was no guarantee we'd get to consume them, but it was a grand idea. My special prayer at that time would be, 'Don't let me set off the fire alarm'.

Some of the lessons we learned were to cover up the lovely wooden floor to get some soft flooring and wear comfortable, flat, quiet shoes. Check whether the activity programme of the day was absorbing, and that everyone at some point got a good dose of fresh air out in the grounds. Make sure there were sufficient meals and snacks throughout the day, and a nice warm milky drink in the evening. If someone got up hungry, have the snack ready. Don't get into a debate about whether it's appropriate to be eating in the night. Usually, after a small snack if it was served up quick enough, we found people got back into bed. We found that when someone tried to persuade them not to turn the night into a day, and tried to guide them back to bed against their wishes, night did in fact become day. It was pointless. My motto—go with the flow as long as it's safe to do so.

There are many variations with beds now, and it really is a case of trial and error. Serious hazards are present in the use of many bed-side designs, which can trap limbs, and can have the effect of frightening people who can't see out, so that they attempt to climb over the side and fall. Some feel secure in an ordinary bed with a mattress on the floor in case of falls. We have nursed people on futons, and mattresses on the floor. But there are serious issues around moving and handling, and the risk to the staff getting back injury should be taken care of.

After trying every type of bed with one client, he finally seemed comfortable on a double mattress on the floor knowing he wasn't going to fall any further. But when his wife visited, she was horrified at how indignified it seemed, and she had a point. He loved to throw the covers around the room and it looked very messy. Once he dropped off, nobody dared to go in and straighten up. Where we fell down, I think, was that although we'd discussed the problem with his wife over the phone, we didn't manage to really prepare her before she arrived. That rapport is crucial. It really can be very upsetting to see someone you love so untidy and on the floor.

But the equipment is getting better and better now, and we are able to have some beds tailor-made. Now, I've seen beds for children with moulded Perspex sides that you couldn't trap a limb in and you can see out of. There are no corners to knock against. I do wonder if something like this maybe useful for some people with advanced neurological conditions. Keep up a good rapport with the manufacturer's representatives. I find they tend to love a challenge. Show them around and let them get to know your clients. A good comfortable adjustable chair can allow for naps in the day between the activities, and this can help to stop over-tiredness developing.

Some people find that hammocks are very comfortable. They go with the movement of chorea, whereas beds are uncomfortable, offering resistance. As I say, trial and error. And be prepared for limited success at times. If all else fails, you may have to consult the doctor regarding medication. Used skillfully, carefully monitored, this can be very helpful, but should not be a first resort. Drugs that affect the central nervous system can sometimes introduce more problems than they were intended to resolve unless used judiciously.

Dying

Once you have got to know your client, your nursing plan will become more and more individualised. It will be changing constantly in response to the changing evaluation and reassessment of the problems you had to work with the client to overcome through the course of these advanced stages of neurological disease. Dying, for all of us is inevitable of course, but for people with advanced neurological conditions and their families it is more than abstract. It is a long process faced by them in their daily lives.

You will be playing an important role in that process, by giving time, and listening to fears and concerns to practical and spiritual matters, working with the person you are caring for. You will also help tie up loose ends where possible, and to come to terms where this will not be possible. Perhaps he or she had wanted to share beliefs with you or express doubts. Maybe you helped to communicate between the individual and the family. There are many ways in which you might have helped in the process of dying without realising.

You must have helped to bring about the maximum comfort possible. At times, you must have been exasperated, even infuriated by the irrational behaviour that can occur in neurological deterioration. That's because you got involved. So you should feel good about that, and take time out to congratulate yourself, and remind your colleagues of the great work that they are doing.

It feels good when the team supports each other because it's going to be hard when the client you have come to know pretty intimately, passes on. No doubt as a team, you've done your best to establish his or her wishes, and liaise with loved ones or an advocate.

Towards the final stages, movement problems such as chorea often tend to settle down, and there can be increased muscular rigidity. Very gentle passive exercise directed by a physiotherapist maybe helpful. Gentle hand massage directed by a therapeutic masseuse or aromatherapist maybe calming also. Good mouth care is essential. Hygiene and care to avoid complications such as pressure sore development by changing position and good use of appropriate mattresses, and the input where necessary of a tissue viability specialist. Generally, at this stage, what nurses know about how to nurse any dying person applies.

Choices may have to be made. Nutrition and hydration are important factors. But how aggressively will it be appropriate to provide these, if swallowing is impaired and oral intake is leading to aspiration is questionable. Ethical choices about the appropriateness or otherwise of tube feeding may have to be addressed, and it is very helpful if they were considered and discussed with the patient and family before the condition became so advanced.

Another issue is whether the person would wish to donate brain tissue for research purposes. Cultural factors can play an important part. To some, the idea of having the brain removed after death would be unthinkable, while to others, it is a gesture of hope for the next generation. It can be seen as a way of living on and an altruistic gift. Maybe there haven't been many opportunities to be the giver of gifts in the family for a long time. It is a good idea to build up a good enough rapport early on, so that long before death is on the visible horizon, a discussion about these wishes can be entered into.

But there can be practical problems with this. Often, there are no funds available to process brain donation. Families are often disappointed when their loved one dies and it is not possible to take the brain. The staff need to be informed and be up to date so that they can inform families who are thinking about this.

There are numerous avenues of hope for effective treatments for degenerative neurological conditions. But perhaps the greatest cause of hope in the immediate future is the nursing plan you have created for your client. In the past such a plan was unlikely. Neurological conditions were very often misunderstood, and people whose behaviour for example, became impulsive or aggressive early on in the development of conditions such as HD were not recognised as becoming ill. Some got into fights or stole impulsively and ended up in a prison. It still occurs, but less so. Many others acting in a bizarre way that society couldn't make sense of were in locked areas within large psychiatric hospitals. People who seemed to be drunk and living immoral lives because of what the disease had done to them were very often social outcasts, roaming in the streets and dying alone.

Your nursing plan is a sign of our society's enlightenment. You understand what a disease affecting the brain can do to people, and you are able to see beyond the abnormal movements, the impaired speech, and the spilled food, to the person inside. It's great that your assessment, your plan and the way you implemented the nursing is beyond the hopes and dreams of the past. But because you will now complete the nursing process with your evaluation, the next plan will be built on what has been learned, what went well and what didn't. That gives us all great hope for nursing in the future. A dying person, who has hope, has riches.

It is important for staff to be up to date, with progress towards effective treatments, as changes occur rapidly. The use of the internet for patients and for staff is very helpful in this. At the end of this book is a list of some useful websites.

I would like to relate to you a story about the funeral of a man I knew as Mike. The priest gave a reverent ceremony, but asked if someone from among the nursing staff would mind getting up and saying a few words, as the priest didn't really know Mike very well.

Laura got up hesitantly and said something along these lines:

'Mike came to our nursing home almost three years ago. He had been living on the city streets, and regularly had attended the soup kitchen. Most people seemingly assumed he was drunk, because of his awkward gait and slurred speech. A worker at the soup kitchen got to know him and began to realise that Mike wasn't drinking. The worker knew a nurse who knew a neurologist who agreed to see Mike. Mike wasn't keen to go, and carried on living rough for a while. Then one cold winter evening he didn't show up at the soup kitchen. The worker went to look for Mike, found him and persuaded him to come and stay in a nearby hostel.

When Mike was a little stronger, he was persuaded to visit the neurologist who was good enough to fix another appointment. The neurologist recognised the type of movement disorder and had Mike tested for the HD genetic mutation. The test was positive. Mike was referred to our home. Actually, at that time his name was not known. No one could understand anything he said other than 'yes' or 'no'. The staff agreed that he looked like a 'Mike', and as he seemed to respond to it, the name was decided upon.

We don't know whether Mike had a family or whether someone out there was looking for him. Apparently, the 'missing person' advertising had carried his picture for a while, without a response. We don't know what he ever did for a living or what hobbies he may have once enjoyed. But we did find out that he loved loud classical music and he loved port. We concluded that he had once enjoyed some of the good things in life.

What we do know is that Mike was, despite giving off a first impression of being outwardly rough and gregarious, was a true gentleman. At least he was to us. He always expressed gratitude despite not having the words to do it. He never asked for much, but he gave. He gave us a sense of fulfilment. He brought out the best in us. He showed us how to be brave and patient. He had a good sense of humour and gave us a lot of fun, even though he was unable to speak.

Mike was an unknown ambassador for all people with a degenerative neurological disorder. He taught us that even though robbed of the past, left without a voice and deprived of the future, there is much to give and much worth living for, and hopefully he found there was much love to receive.

The home will not be the same without you Mike. Thank you for coming to be with us and for making us better people.'

I think that Mike was an ambassador for many more people than just those who have HD and their families. I believe that so many issues are raised when we care for people with any neurological disease that if we could address them well, we will have learned to provide good nursing for all of those we care for in nursing homes.

Later, the staff team saved up and bought Mike a headstone. The epitaph was the last line of Laura's speech.

PART E
BIG DECISIONS

Can I Carry on Caring at Home?

I once worked in a psychiatric hospital where a lady was admitted for assessment, as her husband had told a social worker of his concerns that his wife was becoming difficult to care for. She seemed to be increasingly disorientated and forgetful, and could not concentrate on washing and dressing or other activities of living. She was up half the night walking about, and so he had to keep getting up also to prevent her from falling down the stairs. She had a tendency to wander out of the garden during the day, onto the road, which was narrow and winding. He was fearful that a speeding driver would fail to spot her meandering. He complained that he was feeling more and more like a goal keeper. Gone were the happy times together. They were replaced by a constant series of rounds of coaxing and catching her and returning her to somewhere safe in the house. 'I'm worn out with it', he told a nurse who visited at the social worker's request.

Listening to the problems, the nurse shared the same concerns about the gentleman's wife's welfare and particularly, her mental health. So she arranged the admission. Let's call the gentleman 'Bill' and his wife 'Mary'. Bill visited Mary twice daily usually around noon and then again at about 7pm. After a week or so, it was established that Mary had dementia, and there were discussions about whether she was fit to carry on being cared for at home by

Bill, or whether she might need to be admitted to a nursing home for her safety. Perhaps Bill could manage at home, but would need some home care input, some staff members suggested. Anyway, Bill was invited to a multi-disciplinary meeting, so that his perspective could be considered along with everyone else's. The meeting was arranged for noon, because Bill was always there at that time anyway, and it would save him an extra journey.

This is a tale of shame, I'm afraid. As a nursing team, we had slipped up all over the place and failed miserably. It was long ago, and like another place I will mention from my past, a bit further on in the book, the facility is now closed. It was one of my very early lessons in nursing that was so awful and regrettable. It stayed with me, as I'm sure it did with my colleagues. Basically, we just paid no attention to the obvious. Oh dear!

When we all sat down for the meeting, Bill hadn't arrived. We thought we'd give him a few more minutes before starting. The phone went. It was accident and emergency at the general hospital. They had admitted Bill, who was discovered lying on the grass beside the road by a passing driver. He was suffering from dehydration and exhaustion. When questioned where he had been heading, he managed to say that he was going to a meeting at the psychiatric hospital concerning his wife who was there. It turned out he'd been making this fifteen mile return journey twice daily since Mary's admission. Every day, after returning from the lunchtime visit, it wasn't long before it was time to set off again for the evening visit.

We hadn't noticed the exhaustion. We hadn't asked him how he was getting to and from the hospital. Well, everyone thought someone else had asked things like that. Perhaps the way he looked to us hadn't changed because he'd always been exhausted due to his pervious, at-home routine of running around after Mary. We were shocked not as much by what had happened to Bill, as by our own stupidity and failure. And this was deeply distressing. Every working day, you pull together as a team to do right, and you overlook what is staring at on in the face—a poor man desperately in need of help, giving out stark and clear indications of not being able to cope, and so used to being pushed and stretched way beyond capacity, that the impossible walking challenge didn't seem appropriate to mention.

Why would he think anyone would do anything about it? After all, no one had stepped in to help so far. We were assessing the patient, Mary, but not Bill, the carer. Bill wouldn't have been able to tell you how long he'd been a carer. To do that, he'd have to work out when it was that he'd been looking after May due to her neurological condition. But couples do tend to help each other as a part of their normal life. Her reliance on him to worry about her, and keep a constant eye upon her, lose sleep and intervene with ordinary activities of living would have crept up insidiously, fluctuating in degree over years, and looking back, he wouldn't be able to identify a start date for taking on the role. It's a role that carers tend to take on as a matter of duty. Usually, no one asks formally if they would be prepared to accept it, or teaches them how to go about it.

Mary was placed into a suitable nursing home, where she was regarded not as having 'mental health' or 'psychiatric' problems, but as having a degenerative neurological condition. Accompanied by a staff member, she visited Bill each day in hospital till he recovered. Oh, the awful irony of it.

I have encountered many other memorable occasions when it has turned out that the carer for someone with a neurological disorder was having to deal with much more than seems humanly possible before the professional services acknowledged the problem, even though the signs or circumstances made it obvious that intervention was called for much earlier.

I'll give another example. After a day of managing a nursing home for young people with neurological disorders, I got home fairly late in the evening and sat with my wife to enjoy some tea and watch a bit of TV. At around 10pm, the phone went. It was a social worker who had first rung the nursing home and had been re-routed by staff, because she was persistent. She had taken up a new post after the previous social worker had re-located somewhere else. At around 8pm, she had responded to an emergency call from a 17 year old girl, let's say 'Maria', looking after her father, we'll call 'Ted', who had Parkinson's disease.

Maria had been looking after her dad for several years as he deteriorated. Mum had left home before this and was no longer in touch. Initially, Maria had fitted the caring role around school and then around a daytime job. But as Ted began to need more and more daytime input with washing and dressing, eating and getting to the toilet, this became more unworkable. So Maria had found a job working night shifts at a factory. It allowed her to look after Ted all day, then tuck him up in bed, and go off to do the shift. During this time she had the input from a social worker who had now moved on, and had often explained that it was all too much and that she couldn't cope. But the social worker had consistently attempted to reassure her, saying that Maria shouldn't worry, she was coping very well and was 'a star'. Maria particularly resented being called a star and complained that 'I'm not brilliant. I'm just ordinary, and I can't cope'. To which the previous social worker would reliably repeat, 'Yes you can. You're a star'.

On several evenings as Maria was about to set off for work, there were problems with her father's care, and she had needed to stay with him and sort it out. She'd turned up late a few times and had missed a couple of shifts altogether. The boss had warned her that if she missed another, she'd be sacked. There were no other nearby factories to turn to, and she could not possibly afford to lose the income that they both relied on. So on this particular evening when she found herself changing soiled sheets instead of getting off to work, she had called the social worker's emergency line. The new social worker didn't see a 'star' who was 'doing great'. She saw a young girl who had lost her youth. A boy at the factory had asked Maria out and she had replied 'I'd love to, but I can't have dates, I can't have a life, I have a father with Parkinson's disease.'

Maria had insisted that having changed the sheets she was going to go to work. But Ted had developed a new habit of getting up at night and falling. He would be vulnerable, but Maria reasoned the greater risk to them both would be that of a loss of income.

So, the social worker had got hold of me to ask me to come out and assess whether we could take Ted to the home. When I saw the situation, I agreed some make-shift amendments to our procedure for admissions with the social worker, which normally took some time and involved more professionals. I got Ted into the car (he was willing and keen to come) and by midnight, Ted was in bed at our nursing home; and Maria was at work, and able to tell her boss that she'd found a solution to her time-keeping and absence problems.

Maria couldn't cope, and though the services had known this for a long time, she was left having to cope. Bill couldn't cope, and we had all the information to make that so clear. But he also was left having to cope. So many carers are left coping in unmanageable circumstances, and these days it shouldn't be happening.

This isn't meant to overlook the fact that many do cope well and enjoy a caring role, with the back-up of very good and well-organised support services. It can be a rewarding and satisfying role, and for many people, gives life an added, meaningful sense of purpose and quality and a reason to be.

But, with regard to people who may not have sufficient support, what can save them from falling through society's safety net? Support will vary internationally, and some cultures seem generally better placed than others to support people within an extended family network. But there should be systems to ensure provision, and to make it easy for a person who has found themselves carrying the responsibility of caring for an adult with a neurological disorder, to get help to clarify what they can and can't cope with at home, and whether they do need to start plans to seek a nursing home placement. In the UK, for example, everyone who is regularly giving substantial care to a person over 18 is entitled to request a 'carers assessment' from social services.

In this context, there is no definition of either 'substantial' or 'regular'. So it is left to the judgement of the carer working with the social worker to consider the specific circumstances. The social worker is expected to consider what services are available that could make life easier for the carer and the person being cared for, and where appropriate, help the carer to access the resources.

So, carers are advised to make a list of factors that need to be considered in their assessment. They should note whether they get sufficient sleep; whether their health is affected by caring, and whether they get breaks or must be with the person constantly. They should not compromise on important aspects of leisure and social activities they would like to pursue but are missing because of caring, and whether the role interferes with other interests such as education or not.

However services work in your own location, you need to make your situation well known to health and social care professionals and get help to work out how the pressure can be taken from your shoulders when it is too much and in any case, to give you breaks. Even if you enjoy caring, it is in the interests of the care professions that you are able to carry on, and so they should be very glad to support you. But there may well come a point where what is expected of you as a carer at home is just too much. You may need help to recognise it, so always keep in touch with service providers, and insist that there is a regular carer's assessment, so that you all do recognise if and when the pressures become too great. If you don't look after yourself, and the services don't adequately look after you, you won't be able to care well for your loved one, even with the best of intentions.

If you can't care at home, it is no failure, though for many family members, I know it can feel like failure. Be honest and realistic with yourself. It's not right that your own life and interests should be lost because of your role. If the time for a nursing home placement has come, it is because of the deteriorating condition, not because you are letting anyone down. Look after yourself!

Choosing a Nursing Home

I have frequently referred to a situation where care is being delivered in a nursing home. The decision that a person with a degenerative neurological condition has reached a point where care at home is no longer the best option and that admission to a nursing home is appropriate is surely among the most significant events in anyone's life. For some, it maybe a catastrophic change, defining the loss of all that has been important—home, family, independence... There can be an angry reaction to a sense of betrayal by loved ones who for some unfathomable reason seem to have colluded with professionals to agree that everything the person concerned has held dear, must be taken away.

In such situations, family members often suffer enormous guilt. There maybe grief over the loss they feel, for the loss of the way life used to be and of the person they knew who may have changed almost beyond recognition.

For every case like this, there are much happier scenarios surrounding nursing home admission. Many families have seen the situation developing over time. They have had good professional support, and the person with the neurological diagnosis has been able to foresee the need for the admission and has worked with the family and professionals to choose a suitable home and make arrangements for the day when it comes. This has to be preferable, and is more likely to be achieved where open discussions between family members including the person with the condition and the professional team are fostered. Honesty about the diagnosis and the likely implications is important from the early days of recognising that there is a health problem.

Acceptance of a home and smooth settling in can be helped if the environment and the people there are familiar. And so, where possible, for some, a graduated admission can be a good way to go. This could mean being admitted for a week initially, to give the carer a respite break. Then some more short admissions like that, so that the person is familiar with the people and surroundings, prior to eventually moving in. A plan like this needs to be started long before the situation at home becomes unmanageable, and so requires forward planning.

But how do you know what is a good home? At the time of writing, the authority that registers and inspects care homes in my own country, the UK, is the Care Quality Commission. There has been a succession of changes regarding the name and organization of those responsible for this task in the country over the last decade or so, it may change again. Currently they can be found at http://www.cqc.org.uk

Depending where you are, you may have a similar body with these responsibilities. In this case, the web site is very user-friendly and it can be easy to find homes in the category you are looking for. For example if you click on 'Find Care Services' and then 'Social Care Services' you can then select whether you are looking for a home that offers nursing, or care without nursing. You can select dementia, or physical disability, or sensory impairment, old age and other categories- individually, or tick several of the categories if, say the person has dementia and physical disabilities and mental health problems, for example.

As an option, you can tick the star rating you require. The rating awarded to homes by the Care Quality Commission is explained simply. You can then scroll through homes and when you see a possible candidate, click on the name and you will see a summary description and can read the report from the last inspection. Personally, I have to say, I wouldn't consider any home listed as 'poor'. But I wouldn't rule out those who achieved 'adequate' or 'good' ratings. I would certainly consider those who receive an 'excellent' rating, but I'm still going to have an open mind. The rating tells me how they seemed to be performing on the day of the inspection. Was that a normal day? I don't know and will try to check, if I'm interested in considering the home as an option.

Those who didn't quite seem 'excellent' may have a problem identified. I would read the report carefully. If I wanted to consider a home, I would arrange to visit. Some say, go unannounced, to see things as they are when you're not expected. Personally, I understand that logic, but I wouldn't do it. One reason is that it is someone's home, and I hope no stranger will visit my home unexpected and expect to be allowed in and look around. It's just my personal view.

I'd make the arrangement with the manager. Aren't I scared that it will all seem excellent, but they're putting on a show? Well, maybe, but I doubt it. If the manager insists on staying with us, and only showing us a very guided tour, I may well start to suspect there's something to hide. If I'm finding that as I go to different areas, I'm speaking freely with various staff members and residents, with the manager happy to take a back seat, I'll assume the manager has confidence in what I will see and hear. I find the idea of some sort of act in these circumstances difficult to believe. If the manager doesn't have a good grip of the way the home runs, I'm sure he or she couldn't get everyone to be consistent even on a short planned visit.

I would be checking out if the people seem friendly—staff and residents. I would ask one or two residents what they've been doing today or yesterday. I would note any unpleasant smells such as urine which can raise questions about hygiene. I would check what food is on offer.

How spacious and accessible do rooms seem to be? Do residents seem generally content? I would tell a junior member from the staff what the diagnosis is and ask if they know much about it, and whether they think this would be a good choice of home. If they said yes, I would ask why? What does it have to offer someone like me (or my relative, whoever this quest is for)? If a junior member demonstrates some understanding of the kinds of things about the home and the staff and fellow residents that maybe helpful for a person with the particular diagnosis, I am likely to become quite interested.

Senior staff need the knowledge also, but the trouble is, it's often the more junior members who spend most time helping residents with daily activities of living. They don't need to know much about the condition itself. But if they know the problems I (or he or she, whoever this is for) might experience in trying to sleep, wash, dress, eat, socialise and what might he helpful, that is a very good sign of the way the home runs.

I would make several visits. Soon I won't be a stranger any more, and if they've made me feel welcome, it won't seem rude to turn up one time unannounced.

If the report identified a problem or two, it wouldn't put me off a home that seemed good on my visits. But I would then ask the manager and some staff members what is happening about the identified problems. If I get consistent satisfactory answers, I'll be pleased with that. I would also ask at an 'excellent' rated home, what is happening to maintain the standard and to carry on improving.

Perhaps among the most deciding factors for me, would be recommendations from a happy resident and their family.

Tricky Ethics in Neurological Care

When we are involved in caring for people with a degenerative neurological condition, especially in the advanced stages, we tend now and then to be faced with difficult ethical decisions. Some of the issues that can arise are so controversial, that they become hotly debated through local, national and international media.

As I write this section, it is not long at all since legal history was made in the United Kingdom by a woman named Debbie Purdy who has Multiple Sclerosis and won a battle to have the law on 'assisted suicide' clarified. She wanted to know whether her husband would be prosecuted if he were to help her to end her life by accompanying her to a clinic in Switzerland, where she would be assisted to end her life.

Currently in the UK as in many countries around the world, assisting someone to commit suicide is illegal. There are four places where it is allowed —Oregon, Belgium, Netherlands and Switzerland. Switzerland is the only country where there is no stipulation that a physician must be involved. The other locations require the involvement of two physicians. However, in Switzerland in practical terms, a doctor does need to be present because a medical certificate is required to identify a 'hopeless or terminal' condition before the lethal drugs are administered.

Switzerland has opened up this facility to foreigners and so in recent years has become a place where many people from around Europe and some Americans who wish to end their life at a time under their control, have headed towards.

Many partners, other family members or close friends wanting to support a terminally ill person who decides to go off to Zurich to have their life ended by medical intervention face a serious dilemma. Knowing that they will be accompanied and supported, the person might choose to wait until their condition leaves them dependent and quite disabled. If they know they are not going to be accompanied though, they may have to go much sooner, while independent. This would mean dying alone with strangers, rather than surrounded by loved ones, and giving up life earlier than they really wish to.

And those loved ones may be prevented from going and supporting the person's final voluntary act for fear that they will be regarded as criminals, and arrested on their return home. Many loved ones maybe willing to risk that, but the person wanting to die might not want to put them in that position, and so might insist on going alone. The difficulties associated with this dilemma are compounded by the uncertainty of not knowing whether in fact going to Zurich to help the terminally ill person to the clinic to die is against the law.

Debbie Purdy has brought this uncertainty to a head by winning the right to have the law clarified. She of course hopes the clarification will mean that her husband can go with her to Zurich when the time feels right, without fear of prosecution, and that this will pave the way for others. But a GP Dr Michael Irwin, who has accompanied people to the 'Dignitas' clinic in Zurich, and who was arrested for helping someone financially to go, according to The Independent (2nd August, 2009), believes the clarification may go the other way and make it more likely that people assisting someone to get to Zurich to end their life will be prosecuted.

Some people feel convinced that the law should allow assisting people to Zurich, and for some it should go further and save people the journey and allow assisted suicide in the UK (in Debbie Purdy's case) or wherever the person resides.

Many other people feel that the law shouldn't allow anyone, anywhere to help someone commit suicide.

We wait to see the outcome, but so much for the legal problem. What about the ethics? What is the morally right decision to make about assisting someone to commit suicide? Is it an absolute or is it an issue that can be right in some circumstances and wrong in others? Should we be concerned with what is best for the individual, or should we worry about what would happen to others if we step onto the 'slippery slope'? The 'slippery slope' argument might be that if we allow assisted suicide because we think it should be a matter of choice for those who can freely decide, others may begin to feel pressure to make that decision.

They may feel that their condition is making them a burden on others, so they ought to go to the clinic. Or they maybe persuaded by family members who are waiting to inherit their estate. If week by week the estate is slipping away to pay for nursing care, I wonder how many people would feel that society, without saying so 'expects' them to opt out.

Some people may hold that none of these matters are the fundamental issue. They may feel that life is sacred, and that therefore suicide is inherently wrong, regardless of considerations like free choice or slippery slopes.

You might argue that these debates about what is right and what is wrong ethically are hopeless, even pointless. You'll never get to the right answer, because there isn't one, everyone has their own view. That maybe true, but somehow, we have to make decisions. If someone with an advanced neurological condition asked you, their carer or nurse, to help them end their life, would you? Leaving the law to one side for a moment, would your conscience permit? Even if you thought the person was making a wrong choice, would you be happy to help because it was their choice? To just say 'that's a tough one' 'there's no right answer' and sit on the fence might be becoming for many, an unaffordable luxury.

That's just one issue—assisted suicide. Note that we have not discussed 'euthanasia' or 'mercy killing'. No doubt more contentious in that someone is killed by another, rather than assisted to kill themselves.

There are many other difficult issues that may force us to make ethical decisions in our role as a carer or a nurse for someone with advanced neurological disease. Consider some of the many dilemmas presented by the availability of genetic testing for an inherited condition such as Huntington's disease (HD).

In the section on HD, a scenario is mentioned where a female partner of a man who is at risk of inheriting HD from his parent, is pregnant and wants to have the child genetically tested for the genetic mutation that causes HD. The advice to seek genetic counselling is given in that section. But let's briefly consider some potential ethical dilemmas this situation could pose.

What is the reason for offering a test for the HD genetic mutation for a developing child in the womb? Well, there is an assumption that if the result is positive, a termination will be offered and accepted. At present there is no treatment for this condition that could change the outlook for the baby if born with the mutation- he or she would be destined to develop HD at some time, probably in midlife.

You could argue that the result would be just useful for some mothers or couples to know. They could prepare themselves better. But in reality this situation is avoided. The testing of children under the age of 18 is strongly discouraged. It is widely held that a person should be an adult, old enough to make an informed decision, taking into account the implications of their status being known. The rare exceptions might include for example, if a child at risk is showing signs of juvenile HD, in which case a neurologist may suggest a 'confirmatory' test which could be helpful.

Generally then, the status of someone under 18 at risk of HD is felt to be best unknown. So, the idea that a child might be tested while in the womb and then born is also strongly discouraged.

This situation is bound to be uncomfortable with some while seeming perfectly logical to others. While practical, for many people it begs the question, 'Are we suggesting that it is better for people who are destined genetically to develop HD not to live?' Of course, people who end up getting HD, as people who have accidents or develop any other condition later in life can live as good and meaningful a life as anyone else. So surely it would be wrong to suggest such a thing. For many other people of course, the situation doesn't beg this question at all. It merely offers individual mothers or couples the means to facilitate their own individual choice about how to deal with their own current predicament.

That is an ethical dilemma, where there can be controversy regarding what is 'right' morally.

Another issue raised by this scenario is the father's right to choose for no one to have knowledge of his own genetic status.

If the baby is tested positive for HD, then clearly, the father has the genetic mutation and will develop the disease. If the mother argues for her right to know the child's status, and the father insists on the right to keep his own status unknown, whose rights should take precedence? You may feel that you can answer that one readily, but what is your rationale? Do you have a logical way of working out the right way forward if the rights of two people clash? Are there a third person's rights to consider here? Can the child who isn't born yet be said to have rights already?

Another issue that is sensitive and can provoke enormous anxiety and force difficult choices is 'tube feeding'. This has been briefly referred to in the earlier sections (see under 'Huntington's Disease'; 'Multiple Sclerosis', 'Eating and Drinking' and 'Dying'). It's another topic that has generated some high profile controversial decisions. For example, Leslie Burke, who was 43 when diagnosed with Friedreich's Ataxia back in 2003 turned to the British courts for assurance that in the future when his condition leaves him unable to communicate, and he cannot eat and drink by mouth, doctors will provide him with nutrition and hydration via a tube into his stomach. This is known as 'PEG' feeding, or 'Percutaneous Endoscopic Gastrostomy'.

Initially, the courts agreed that this was his right and he won his case. But the British General Medical Council (GMC) appealed and in 2005 the court decision was overturned. The principle established was that patients cannot dictate to doctors that they must carry out a procedure. Doctors will make the decision at the time. They must take into account the patient's wishes, but also must consider whether it is the right clinical decision at the time and in the current circumstances. Opting out of the procedure on the other hand would be a patient's right.

I have encountered some tricky 'tube feeding' decision-making scenarios while nursing people with advanced neurological conditions. Although, as indicated in earlier sections, it is best to try to address issues such as whether in the advanced stages, the person would want to be tube fed. Often this hasn't happened. Staff for example at a nursing home might begin to report that helping the person with drinks and food is increasingly difficult, and that they fear the person is aspirating; that is, inhaling food and fluid. There is a danger of choking but also, of developing pneumonia, which can easily become the unpleasant cause of death.

In these circumstances a tube is not necessarily the best answer. It is important to involve a speech and language therapist who can assess swallowing and can offer advice on food texture and thickening of drinks to a 'nectar' 'single cream' or other suitable consistency using thickening products. They can arrange a 'video fluoroscopy' so that problems with swallowing can be seen via an x-ray film, which helps with a thorough assessment. I mentioned in the 'Eating and Drinking' section that I have found that it also helps staff members to understand the right amount to load onto a spoon and how long to wait before offering another spoonful, because they are better able to visualize what the problem is with swallowing.

Taking the trouble to ensure an environment conducive to eating and drinking helps greatly (quiet and predictable) and so does getting the right posture by choosing a good chair and adjusting it appropriately, until swallowing is easier. Smaller, more frequent meals or snacks are often more manageable than waiting, becoming hungry, and then trying to desperately gulp down a large meal.

But despite these efforts, many people reach the point where the only way to receive nutrition and hydration without aspirating or choking is via a tube. But is it appropriate? Some people feel that this just prolongs the agony, when nature would more kindly end life and the suffering more naturally without the tube. Hopefully, the family members as well as the health professionals will work together, not to agree what they think is best so much (although that's important too), but to agree on what they believe the person's choice is or would be if they were able to express it.

Often by this stage, speech is badly affected also, and so it becomes difficult for the patient to get across to staff what their wishes are about having or not having a tube inserted. There is often frustration all around, as staff struggle to get the person to make an informed choice and convey it to them. Often, staff members become divided about what they believe the person wants or is trying to tell them. Once it is fitted, the tube can irritate the person and they might begin pulling at it. Some will think that is confirmation it wasn't wanted, while others disagree and feel that it cannot prolong life beyond when the brain and body begin 'shutting down', but that it would be cruel to allow death without basic care such as food and fluid.

Although it is often easier in these situations if the person has previously indicated their choice about tube feeding either verbally or in a written 'living will' (as with other end of life decisions), that isn't always the case. A lady in our care, let's call her Brenda, had progressive Multiple Sclerosis or 'MS'. She told us on one lunch time as she cut into her meat. 'You see Madge over there, having her food cut for her... when I get to that stage, I don't want you to cut it up, I'd rather go without; it will be time to let nature run it's course and allow me to die while I still have some dignity.

Brenda knew that Madge also had progressive MS, and Brenda couldn't see any dignity in having food cut up for her. Later though, Brenda did reach a point where she couldn't manage to cut her food. She asked for it to be cut, and no one reminded her that she had previously insisted that she would refuse this to happen.

Everyone found it easy to agree that the current choice she was making was more important than the choice she made while the situation was still only hypothetical.

Then Brenda told us. 'You see Madge over there, with her food softened... when I get to that stage, I won't have it, I will go without'. The time came when she couldn't manage food unless softened and she readily accepted it. But she said, 'You see Madge, with her food liquidized... I won't have that, you mustn't give it to me when I get to that stage'. But the stage arrived and Madge asked for it to be liquidized.

Then Madge said. 'You see Madge there, having her food and fluids through a tube into her stomach... I don't want that, when I reach that stage don't give it to me.' These wishes were documented by the nurses. The time came when Brenda could no longer manage food or fluids safely any way other than via a tube, despite the best efforts of the staff team. By this time, Brenda could no longer speak, and it really was difficult to know when she was trying to indicate a 'yes' or a 'no' through sounds and gestures that she made.

The team were very divided and so were the family members who were invited to help staff reach a decision about what Brenda wanted. Some said, 'She clearly indicated that when she got to this stage she did not want a tube inserted'. Others pointed out, 'Yes that's true. But you know as each situation became a reality she moved her own goal posts'.

We did eventually reach a unanimous decision; not about what we thought was best, but about what we thought Brenda's choice was. Brenda did get the tube inserted, but we were never sure that we had interpreted her wishes correctly.

So, is there a better way to go about it? It is always necessary to involve the individual as far as they are able to take part, and where appropriate next of kin or an advocate, in the decision process. Also, you need to gather the views of the relevant professionals. These must include a speech and language therapist, a dietician, and a surgeon being asked to perform the operation. Clearly if the client is not a good candidate for anaesthesia, or for some other reason is not suitable for surgery, the decision is easier to reach.

In some cases we have involved a clinical psychologist and a psychiatrist. These have helped us to work out whether the person can understand and is competent to make an informed decision themselves. If a view was made known formally or informally previously, we can gain help to assess whether that is still the wish now that the problem is real and current. The clinical ethics committee can be consulted for advice and guidance if necessary. Despite all this consultation and tending to start the process some six months ahead of the problem becoming a crisis, I have never found reaching a decision easy. To make matters worse, I have often found that even in a room full of family members and professionals, I have been able to easily swing the majority view from one position to another, while trying to outline the potential benefits and disadvantages of each. Colleagues have told me too that they have experienced this feeling and that they worry about it.

Of course, as indicated above, I must emphasise that as far as possible, we try to discuss these issues with clients and families before it becomes impossible to give informed consent. But there are still difficulties in knowing whether the choices made earlier are still what the person wants later on. Debates like this have led to arguments in the UK, surrounding the use of 'living wills' and the introduction of the 'Mental Capacity Act' (2005Act). This Act is underpinned by a set of five key principles. I outlined them in the earlier section on 'Maintaining Safety under the sub-heading

'Preventing falls / damage limitation'. I feel it is worth spelling them out again here, to help with thinking about how they might apply in the context of decisions about tube feeding.

They are :

1. **A presumption of capacity :** Every adult has the right to make his or her own decisions and must be assumed to have capacity to do so unless it is proved otherwise.

2. **The right for individuals to be supported to make their own decisions :** People must be given all appropriate help before anyone concludes that they cannot make their own decisions.

3. Those individuals must retain the right to make what might be seen as eccentric or unwise decisions.

4. **Best interests :** Anything done for or on behalf of people without capacity must be in their best interests.

5. **Least restrictive intervention :** Anything done for or on behalf of people without capacity should be the least restrictive of their basic rights and freedoms.

Is it a problem, if professionals do sometimes feel that they are making the decision despite 'being seen to' go through appropriate processes? I don't know. Often the individual and the family seem to prefer to be told something will be a better choice, than be made to keep mulling over all the options. I think that the difficulty in getting people to come down strongly in favour or not reflects the many ways the choice can be viewed. No one wants to prolong a difficult death. But if life can have a greater quality during the last years, of course it is a great choice. Of course, it's usually only with hindsight that we are able to judge whether it has been a good decision. My thoughts have tended to be that we got it right. I have known many people who had a tube for years and enjoyed what seemed to be an optimum quality of life given the circumstances. Others have had many problems with the tube. We can only do our best.

Even if it does seem (I stress that this is nothing more than an impression) as though others in the process didn't always actively share the choice, they are empowered in that they were party to the process. They know what happened, and by being quiet, probably were demonstrating trust in the judgement of professionals. Surely that's not a problem? I wonder what your view will be.

Confidentiality

Confidentiality about the diagnosis can be another very tricky ethical issue. A gentleman we will call Joe had Huntington's disease. He had begun to act strangely in midlife, seeming selfish and impulsive, and often acting angrily if he didn't get his way. He left home, leaving his wife and five children to get on with life. These 'symptoms' as they turned out to be, appeared before the movement disorder was noticeable in Joe's case, and so it wasn't apparent to the family that he was becoming ill. He just seemed to have become unreasonable and inconsiderate.

Years later, he was clearly ill and the movement disorder was obvious. He couldn't care for himself and was admitted to a nursing home. The family by now had lost touch... although, he had apparently sent them a letter at some point, telling them that he was unwell with Parkinson's disease. It was documented at the nursing home that Joe did not want the family to know he had Huntington's, and wished to protect them from the knowledge that his children (well- they were grown up now) were at a 50% risk of inheriting his awful condition.

Joe deteriorated and was unable to speak when one day three of his children made a visit to the nursing home, each with their partners. They tried communicating with their Dad, but found it upsetting, and couldn't work out what responses he was trying to make. Then they asked to see the nurse in charge of the shift, Angela. They asked Joe's diagnosis, and explained that they suspected it wasn't Parkinson's disease as they had been led to understand. Some distant relatives they had come into contact with had suggested Joe might have a condition that the children were at risk of developing and passing on to their children, but they didn't know what it was called.

Angela was a newly qualified nurse, and was new to working at the home, and she truthfully told Joe's visitors that she didn't know Joe's diagnosis. It was the weekend, and she promised that on Monday when the manager returned, she would contact them. When the manager did return, she told Angela that it was Joe's right to keep his diagnosis to himself. Angela should say that she cannot disclose any information to the family about Joe's diagnosis, as it is confidential information. Angela was uncomfortable with this. She contacted a Huntington's Family Counsellor, who explained that she could only approach the family if they contacted her first. Angela couldn't tell the family to do that, without giving away that the condition was Huntington's disease as the contact details were those of a Huntington's support organisation.

Angela contacted her nursing union, and her nursing professional body. They both advised the same as her nurse manager not to break the confidentiality, saying that Joe had the right to keep his diagnosis a secret. They both warned that Angela would risk disciplinary action if she broke confidentiality, and could be struck off the nursing register for unprofessional behaviour. That means she would lose her job and would not be allowed to practice anywhere as a nurse. She rang the family and said that she had no information about Joe's diagnosis, and that they would have to rely on what Joe had told them.

But a couple of evenings later, after finishing a shift at the home, Angela was half way home when she pulled up in a lay-by, and sat contemplating the situation. One of the couples had said they were planning a family and said that if there were any implications for children they might bring into the world, known by nurses, then they should be told so that they can factor this into their decisions about having children.

One of Joe's daughters had said that two of her brothers were in prison, both having got into trouble for impulsive behavior—taking things not belonging to them and getting into fights. This seemed out of character, and their sister was worried that it was the same impulsive behaviour she had seen in her father when she was very young.

Angela turned the car around and drove to Joe's daughter's house. She got the three couples who had visited Joe together, and told them Joe's diagnosis, and explained the implications for the family. They were very upset and distressed by the news, but were grateful to Angela for telling them. Angela visited the prisons where Joe's two sons were, and informed them. They asked her to make it known to the prison authorities, and they requested genetic testing for Huntington's. It was confirmed that both were showing early signs of the condition, and they were released into care, their 'crimes' now being understood as the result of a devastating illness and not their fault.

Angela never did get into any trouble for this. She informed her manager about what she had done and documented all the events, but she heard no more about it, except that the family kept in touch with her for many years.

What do you think? Did Angela act unprofessionally? What would you have done in her position? How should she have weighed up what was the right thing to do?

Duty of Care

Mrs. Daley was fastidious throughout her life. She was house proud, and was always seen well groomed and 'made up'. Since she developed dementia and went to live in a nursing home this concern with her cleanliness and personal presentation diminished. When staff members tried to persuade her to have a wash, she told them to leave her alone, and similarly when they offered to help her to dress in fresh clothing, she insisted in sitting in her nightwear.

In an effort to keep in accordance with Britain's 'Mental Capacity Act' (2005), the staff team decided to resist being too paternalistic, by insisting on their own standards. They started from the assumption that Mrs Daley was competent, and had the capacity to make her own choices. They consulted a psychologist and a psychiatrist, who both reached the conclusion that Mrs Daley understood the consequences of poor hygiene and the potential social impact of remaining unkempt. She agreed that if she were to become soiled or incontinent of urine, she would accept a bath and change of clothing.

But she couldn't see what was wrong with being a bit scruffy and dirty, which was her choice. Family members who visited however, were not at all happy. They demanded to know how and why staff could be so neglectful as to leave her sitting with food down her front. Her hair was tangled and she was generally bedraggled. This didn't fit with her normal way of life. They were disgusted that staff used the excuse that this was her choice. Of course, they reasoned, she wouldn't make a choice like that if she was able to see herself. She had told them all before she was admitted, that she didn't mind going into a nursing home, but had asked them to stick up for her if she wasn't able to do so for herself, and if she wasn't being cared for properly.

Mrs. Daley's son told the nurse in charge, she may say no to being washed and dressed, but she would easily be persuaded, and your duty of care is more important than your respect for her choice- especially when her real choice, if she had all her faculties, would be to be well presented as she always has been'. The nurse replied 'I realise this is upsetting and I'm so sorry about it. But it's not right for us to insist or persuade anyone in our care to do what they don't want to do. She obviously used to like being tidy and dressed up. But she does have the right to change her mind and have a new outlook.

Who would you say is right?

Making Ethical Decisions

Ethics are the rules or the principles that help to determine the right conduct in a given situation or set of circumstances. They apply to specific groups of people such as a culture or a profession. So, we may hear of 'Christian ethics' or 'Military ethics'. 'Medical ethics' governing doctors are closely related to 'nursing ethics' but there are differences in emphasis. Both require respect for dignity and equality for example but medical ethics maybe regarded as historically more paternalistic; more ready to assume that the professional may know what is best for the person, while nursing principles traditionally have arguably placed more emphasis on facilitating the person to take control of their own lives and make their own decisions.

These differences don't reflect disagreement about what is right but they do reflect differences in the traditional focus of the two professional roles. Medicine is traditionally about working towards a cure while nursing is about caring. In practice of course, these areas overlap.

Before deciding the 'right' thing to do in a specific situation, it is worth thinking about and becoming aware of any assumptions you might tend to make, perhaps often unconsciously. Sometimes people argue about what is right, and are baffled about why the other person can't see their obvious rational arguments not realising that they are each coming to the topic from a fundamentally different underlying perspective, preventing each other from seeing the other's logic.

So, what are these underlying perspectives? Well, moral theory can be 'rights based', 'duty based' or 'goal based'. Rights based and duty based approaches to ethical decision-making are 'non-consequentialist'. That is, things are inherently right or wrong, and being primarily concerned with what the outcome might be, is missing the point. If it is wrong to lie, then it will always be wrong to lie in any circumstances. It maybe forgivable in some circumstances, for instance, if you lie to protect someone from harm, but in principle it is wrong.

Goal based moral theory on the other hand is concerned with the outcome. Lying maybe wrong in some instances and right in others depending on what will bring about the greatest good. Rights based moral theory as the name suggests, places the emphasis on the right action being to protect people's rights. People have the right to be autonomous, to make their own choices, for example, and the right to dignity, and to equality. In duty based moral theory, the essence of the action gives it its value. If you do your duty, you've done the right thing, even if there is a bad outcome.

Problems come about when one person's rights infringe on another's. Joe, above, may have had the right to confidentiality, not to have his diagnosis disclosed. But his children have the right make informed choices about their future. The choices can only be informed if they are given the information that the nurse, Angela, knows.

Duties may also clash. A nurse like Angela has a duty towards her employer, who pays her to do what her manager asks. There is a duty to her patient and failure in this can be addressed through civil law, in a civil court. She has a duty to the wider public, which can be determined through criminal law, in a criminal court. There is a duty to her profession—to keep to a professional code of conduct. Usually, these areas of duty will be in harmony, but they can clash.

On the positive side, adhering to moral principles based on rights or duties gives consistency and certainty. It is easier to know what is right and what is wrong. Also, it protects individuals, underpinning human rights. You cannot mistreat a person because he or she is a minority, and because your course of action is better overall for most people. And principles are reliable over time, not tending to get 'watered down' just because we meet with difficult situations. But on the down side, we could end up doing things because of principles, unconcerned that actions result in people becoming worse.

Goal based moral theory on the other hand embraces 'utilitarianism'—'the greatest good for the greatest number of people'. The right thing to do depends on what we predict the outcome to be.

So, it might be an individual's right to choose 'assisted suicide'. But duty based principles may indicate that helping someone towards an early death is inherently wrong. A consequentialist might argue that regardless of rights or duties, it is better for these individuals if they avoid the suffering associated with the late stages of illness. But another consequentialist might point out the dangers of stepping onto a 'slippery slope'... if this is allowed, people in future could come under pressure to feel it's a choice they ought to take. If you're fixed on the rights of an individual to make a choice, to end their life at a time and in circumstances suitable to them, the politics of 'slippery slopes' may seem irrelevant.

So, as said, before launching into a decision about what to do, or before arguing with colleagues or friends about what is right, it can be helpful to stop and consider whether you tend to be governed by any of these underpinning positions. Are you primarily concerned with an individual's rights? With your sense of duty, to do what is right? Or with an outcome that is likely to be best for most people? If you are dealing with people who tend to disagree with you, can you work out where they are coming from, regarding these positions?

Understanding how we are driven ethically is helpful and can enable us to understand sometimes, why another person, also caring and keen to do what is best, might not follow our way of thinking. If we can see another person's perspective, we maybe a step nearer to resolving a difficult ethical problem.

But the next step towards a practical solution may require a structured framework to enable us to consider and balance the different aspects of an ethical problem, making sure we have accounted for the different competing factors that need to be considered.

There are a range of suitable frameworks and here, the 'four principles approach' (Beuchamp and Childress, 2001) adopted by the UK Clinical Ethics Network, and used in hospitals and other healthcare settings internationally, is briefly presented.

The four principles to consider are: respect for autonomy, beneficience, non-maleficience and justice.

The principle of respect for autonomy requires that we establish those who have the capacity to make an autonomous decision. We should start from the assumption that people do have this capacity unless there is evidence to the contrary. Given that a person is able to understand the choice and other options, and the consequences of making or not making a particular choice, we should respect the choice the person makes. It may not be the choice that we would make, and it may seem eccentric or even foolish. But this principle is about allowing or even enabling the person to make the choice. If a person does not have the capacity to make an informed choice however, then it is a different matter.

Again, every reasonable effort should be made to try to empower the person to make their own choice. Information may need to be simplified for example. The person may need a bit more time or a quieter environment to make it easier to think about options. If the person really cannot choose, we may need to consult someone who has a lasting power of attorney, and in any case, if we go against the person's expressed wishes, we must be prepared to demonstrate that we are acting in their best interests. That last point leads onto the next ethical principle—beneficience.

The principle of beneficience requires that we do just that; act in a person's best interests, to do them good. We should act in a way, in other words, that benefits the person we are caring for.

The third principle, non-maleficience, requires that we don't do the person any harm. In fact, any intervention might cause some harm. If I was to take Mrs. Daley to the bathroom by subtly persuading her, when she would be happier to continue watching TV in her dirty clothes, she might be upset, and this would be harmful to some degree. On the other hand, if I leave her there, and her family becomes upset because she is unkempt, and this in turn makes Mrs. Daley upset, that maybe harmful also. But the principle is about making sure that any harm is minimized as far as possible and is outweighed by the benefits to the person.

The fourth principle is that of justice. According to this principle, resources, benefits, risks and costs should be distributed fairly.

Let's think about the case of Leslie Oliver again referred to earlier. This is the gentleman with Friedreich's Ataxia, who lost his case in the end when he challenged the British General Medical Council by asking for reassurance that when unable to eat and drink without intervention, he would be tube fed.

Using the four principles approach, how can it be argued that he should not be given this guarantee? Well, regarding autonomy, there was no question about his ability to make his own informed decision in advance. If this were the only principle to consider then, there would be no argument. He should have the intervention because he freely chooses it.

But what about the second principle, beneficience? Will it be in his best interests? Will it benefit him? He argued that it would be in his best interests. Without it he would not have adequate nutrition and hydration and would die. But there maybe an argument that you cannot be sure in advance that this will benefit him when the time comes. He may for example be so ill that he would not be a suitable candidate for a general anaesthetic, or any operation required to insert a tube into his stomach.

And what about non-maleficience? To go ahead and insert the tube if he is not a good surgical candidate may do him harm. There could be skin problems associated with the wound. If he has a low resistance to infection this might increase the likelihood. There maybe psychological harm if by then he is so ill that he no longer wants an intervention to prolong his life, but is unable to communicate his change of wishes. A fairly common example of how people do tend to change their mind when the situation is real rather than hypothetical, is that of a woman preparing to go into labour, who tells the midwife and her partner, 'No matter what I say and how much I scream, don't give me pain relief, I want a natural delivery'. Some of course keep to their original plan, but I equally admire those who respond to the changed circumstances by saying. 'Second thoughts, get me an epidural'.

If Mr. Leslie were to change his mind but could no longer speak to tell anyone and was stuck with the original plan, even though doctors at the time felt pretty sure that he seemed no longer happy about it, they would potentially be doing him psychological harm.

And how about the principle of justice. Is it a fair way to allocate resources to allow people ahead of their time of need, to demand what interventions they wish to have, and to bind doctors by these wishes even though they might not think the intervention is suitable? Arguably not. Perhaps someone tending to adopt a rights based approach to moral principles might have supported Mr. Oliver's stand on the basis that it should be his right to choose how he wants to be treated in the final days of his life. You could say his right to life is even more deserving of support and this would be best served by agreeing to the tube feeding.

On the other hand, someone tending towards a greater concern for a goal based approach, and concerned about consequences might worry that if one person is allowed to pre-order treatment, it will become a trend with doctors having to ignore their own clinical judgment and be governed by pre-determined arrangements. The potential cost to the health service might be enormous, and therefore unjust. Money being spent on dying people, on procedures that may not help and maybe inappropriate, at the cost of resources needed for people who would benefit.

I am not trying to suggest that one of these arguments is more credible than another. I am just trying to demonstrate how becoming familiar with these ethical principles can enable the arguments to be presented in a structured way, so that all aspects and perspectives can be more easily weighed against each other than if they are presented as fairly random ideas.

How about the issue of confidentiality highlighted by the story of the Nurse named Angela and her nursing home resident Joe. Lets see if the four principle framework could have helped Angela to reach her difficult decision in which she chose to go against the advice given by her manager, her nursing union and her professional governing body. Remember that Joe was the man who didn't want his family to know they were each at a high (50%) risk of inheriting his degenerative neurological condition (Huntington's disease) and so he told them he had Parkinson's. He now could no longer speak and the family suspected they might be at risk of something and wanted Angela to tell them what it was.

Regarding autonomy, Joe had made a conscious decision to keep his diagnosis confidential. The problem about rights here is one of Joe's right to confidentiality, and the family's right to know about a condition that has implications for their own futures. You may argue that Joe is Angela's primary concern. It is his rights she is duty bound to guard first and foremost. This wouldn't be to deny that she had a duty of care to Joe's family but would assert that it had to be secondary to her duty to Joe.

Beneficience: Well, Angela might have reasoned that she couldn't really benefit Joe a great deal by either keeping his secret, or by telling it unless she reasoned that he had lied in order to do his family good, but didn't realise that it would do them more good to know the truth. Maybe it does benefit Joe to help his family, even if to do so goes against his expressed wishes. Maybe not. Regardless of this conundrum, Angela believed that she could certainly benefit the family by telling them the truth and giving them the power to make important decisions for their lives.

Non-maleficience: Again, she didn't feel she would harm Joe by telling or not telling the family. But harm could be done to the family, she reasoned, by keeping the truth from them.

Remember that two of Joe's sons would have remained in prison if the authorities hadn't known about their inherited condition and would not have got the care they needed. Anxieties and uncertainties would have persisted and the couples who had visited Joe would have made life choices without knowing their risk status and without specialist support services available to them now.

Justice: Angela felt that she and other health professionals were in possession of knowledge that rightfully belonged to Joe's offspring. The implications of Joe's diagnosis for them were huge, and just as they inherited the disease risk of 50%, they deserve to inherit the knowledge of it. Neither Joe, nor the nurses had the right to keep them in the dark, according to the fairness and equity that are crucial aspects of the justice principle.

No doubt Angela's manager and nursing union and professional governing body could use the same principles to argue for maintaining Joe's confidentiality, but if she was made to give an account of her actions before any hearing, she could do so very much more convincingly by demonstrating her use of a structured approach, than if it appeared she had acted on an impulse. That's the point about making these difficult ethical decisions with a recognised framework. It enables you to be accountable, that is, to give a satisfactory account for your actions or omissions. Nurses are obliged to do so, but anyone in a caring role, formal or informal, would be in a better position if they can justify what they decide to do or not do in this way, even if they only need to justify it to themselves.

So, how can the framework, the four principles, help to resolve the issue about whether a woman pregnant with the child of her partner at risk of HD should be able to have the baby tested in the womb, despite the protests of her partner that his status should not be known?

Regarding autonomy, doesn't the partner have the capacity to make an informed decision to not have his risk status disclosed? Then again, doesn't his partner who is pregnant have the capacity to make an informed decision about whether to bring a child into the world who may or may not have a genetic mutation that would result in a degenerative neurological disease developing probably in midlife? Note that the principles can't answer the argument about whose rights here should take precedence. But they do help to clarify what the argument is. Perhaps the child is the person whose rights should take precedence over both parents in this scenario? But the child is not competent. He or she does not have the capacity to make an informed decision.

I must apologise that this very difficult and sensitive scenario raises issues that maybe painful to consider. If this is a bit close to home, it maybe best to skip the questions I pose in the next couple of paragraphs and seek help from a genetics counsellor, to work through your own personal circumstances rather than worry about generalizations and differences between extreme views that are mentioned below.

If autonomy was a difficult and a complex factor to consider, how about beneficience? And non-maleficence? Whose interests are best served if the child is or is not tested for the HD genetic mutation? Who could be harmed? The father will argue that he will benefit psychologically by not having the child tested. If the child's result is negative, it will not change the father's risk status, he still may or may not have the mutation. But if the child is tested to be positive, then the father will be positive also and will know that at some point the disease symptoms will become evident. He can function better in life meanwhile without having to deal with this news and would be harmed if he had to face it earlier than is necessary.

But the mother of the unborn child can argue that she will benefit by knowing if she is carrying a child who will develop HD or who will not. She might suggest that to bring a child into the world knowing he or she will develop a devastating neurological diagnosis is to harm the child. But there might be an argument that to decide for a child that he or she should not live because of a future illness is to harm the child. Any of us may in the future be ill or have a serious accident or some other awful challenge to face or suffering to endure. If so, are we better off not to live at all? If we take a consequentialist view, what does it say about the value of the lives of people born with the HD genetic mutation? Will it be okay to say that they would be better not to live? Doesn't it seem a little arrogant to write off the value of a life that may focus on what I can do, rather than what I at some point can't do? Having the ability and natural tendency to be able to see everyone's point of view can be a problem. It seems a friendly trait but with regard to having to make decisions, it can be a crippling handicap.

But of course, many would not take a longer term consequentialist view. A rights based approach that considered the pregnant mother's rights as paramount would favour her having the knowledge available to decide what is right for her to deal with, without having to contend with rather hypothetical or theoretical and somewhat vague consequences for the wider population.

Regarding justice, different international cultures and laws will determine in this scenario whose rights are indeed paramount and what is fair. That's if it came down to this. But ideally, the situation would be resolved without having to force any of these issues. A good competent genetics counsellor may have these ethical principles in mind. But using skills to help a couple air their points of view and concerns, maybe able to allow them to reach an amicable joint decision.

Let's pick up one more scenario presented earlier in this section; the one concerning Brenda, who had progressive MS, and told nurses and care staff that she would not want her food cut or have a soft diet or liquidized, when she reached a point where these were necessary. But as she did come to each stage she changed her mind-without acknowledging any contradiction. Then she had told them that she would not accept tube feeding, and as she reached a point where this would be the only way to receive adequate nutrition and hydration, she could no longer speak.

The team were divided if you recall about whether she had changed her mind and now wished to be tube fed, or whether they should honour the request she had made previously.

Again, it is important to emphasise that the ethical principles do not provide answers. They offer structure for the difficult discussions that need to take place. It is important that the discussions in circumstances such as these should involve those directly providing care—experts such as speech and language therapist, psychologist and physician and close family members who can help with determining what Brenda would be likely to choose in the situation if she could make the choice known, and if applicable, the person with the power of attorney.

Regarding autonomy, there is little doubt that Brenda had the capacity to make an informed choice when she said that she would not want tube feeding in the future, and unless it can be proved otherwise this capacity must be assumed. There is not really much of an issue about that. The difficult issue is whether she is now sticking with that same choice or has changed her mind about it in the light of experience. This is because she did have a tendency to change her mind when faced with the reality of changed (though predictable, foreseeable) circumstances, the claim by some staff members that she may have changed her mind now and may wish to be tube fed is reasonable and needs to be considered seriously.

Every reasonable effort should be made to facilitate Brenda to indicate her choice. The use of sign boards can be helpful, and the psychologist maybe able to use expertise to determine whether Brenda is able to express current wishes. The speech and language expert can help to confirm that less invasive measures to provide nutrition and hydration have been adequately attempted and whether tube feeding is clinically appropriate. All who know Brenda and have had a rapport with her can contribute to the discussion about what they might feel she is trying to indicate, if anything, what she understands about her current circumstances, and what she would want to say if she were able to speak.

If some feel that when she indicated her choice earlier, she really could anticipate how she would feel when she got to this situation and therefore did make a fully informed choice, then they should say so, as this would be a crucial factor. If that were to be the case, her choice must be respected. She is opting out of an intervention, not demanding one as was the case with Mr. Oliver.

Beneflcience and non-maleficience: If the autonomy question cannot satisfactorily be resolved, then decisions must be made for Brenda. Will tube feeding benefit her? There will be arguments for and against. It may keep her nourished and hydrated...that can certainly be seen as a benefit. It may prolong her life. Whether that is a benefit or could be seen as harm- prolonging endurance and suffering, is arguable. This may raise questions about her quality of life and satisfaction. If she has not got a good quality of life, can it be improved? Or is dissatisfaction from within, closely tied to her condition so that efforts to improve care and the environment will not alter the fact that she is unhappy to have life extended, some would say by artificial means? (Others might say by necessary, low tech means).

These are the questions that would need to be considered if (only if) the question of Brenda's autonomy was not resolved.

Justice: Is it a fair and equitable use of resources to continue to feed Brenda by inserting a tube and providing costly sustenance on an ongoing basis, when the inevitable course of nature cannot be avoided? Brenda is after all, sadly, going to die. Is there greater justice in allowing this to happen without intervening in such an invasive way, or is it a necessary and justifiable comfort measure, aimed at easing the process of dying rather than at postponing it? These are mixed practical, resource and clinical questions. It may well be just to expend resources if the purpose is comfort, where perhaps it wouldn't be if the purpose were to prolong life.

I know that the above examples don't answer tricky ethical questions that you maybe faced with specifically. But I hope that they give some idea about how your questions can be approached, and how the questions that do need to be answered, with the help of a team, can be identified.

Should We Agree to the Scan?

If the neurologist suggests having a brain scan it will be for a good reason. But the idea of it maybe off-putting for some people and there maybe a feeling that regardless of what can be seen on the scan, it's pointless having it if it only confirms a condition that can't be cured. That is a reaction that can be understood, as is that of a concerned family who think that mum or dad or whichever loved one is being seen by his or her GP (family doctor) or neurologist or perhaps a clinical psychologist or maybe a professional from the mental health team such as a psychiatric nurse or a psychiatrist or who may have seen all of the above, has enough troubles, without the stress of going through tests that in the end may not be helpful.

So, it maybe useful to consider what is involved in brain scanning and what purpose is served with regard to particular suspected neurological disorders.

You will find that a brain scan isn't the first idea that the neurologist will resort to. If a neurological disorder is suspected, the first two things the neurologist will want to do is to get a full medical history and a good picture of the person as a whole.

Let's consider first, someone who raises concerns about some aspects of their cognition. Perhaps there have been recent increasing problems related to memory or organizing the day, preparing lunch or sorting out money. They may have noticed it themselves and reported it to the doctor or concerned relatives or neighbours may have raised the alarm; or perhaps the person is in a nursing or residential care home for elderly people and maybe staff members have notified the professional team that there seem to be changes in these cognitive abilities.

First, the doctor would seek to rule out causes that might be reversible. Depression, vitamin B12 deficiency or a urine infection are examples of problems that can be treated and resolved, but in the mean time can seem to mimic some of the signs associated with cognitive deterioration.

A careful history would be taken to get a picture of what has been the person's normal behaviour and temperament, and a feel for the person's general outlook on life, interests and normal level of sociability. The doctor will try to determine when it was that changes seemed to take place, what these changes were and whether it all happened fairly suddenly or over a long period of time.

Getting this background picture requires skill. If the person's cognition is changing, they may not be able to give a reliable account of the past. If they are afraid of the outcome of the assessment they may, without meaning to, distort the true picture or deny problems that have occurred altogether. Family members also may find it difficult to think clearly about when the problems they have noticed may have started. It can feel sometimes as though you are letting someone you love down by highlighting forgetfulness, or unreasonable behavior or worse, it can feel a bit like making accusations. Perhaps many incidents over time were written off as just normal aging, until things got so unlike the person's character that it had to be admitted that something was wrong. In that case, naturally, it is difficult to look back and pinpoint the time when the pattern of decline we really do associate with aging became a little more significant.

A skilled and experienced health professional can help people feel sufficiently at ease to answer questions openly and give a good account of life before any of the problems are reported, and avoid the situation of feeling like an interview in which people are likely to become anxious about whether they are giving the 'right' answers, or at least, the answers that the professional wants to hear. They need to feel that there are no 'right answers'. It's just a case of getting a good feel for how the person answering sees things.

Skill and experience will also help the doctor know which answers can be taken literally, as reliable facts, and which convey more of an impression of how things are now or may have been in the past. And the impressions we hold can have just as much bearing on our health as any facts can.

This is so important because cognition and mood are so individual. If I get to a good old age and can't remember family birthdays, it's not much of an issue probably. I love them all, but never did remember those dates or organize my diary. I'll catch them in the summer or at a wedding or at Christmas maybe, and we'll have a drink, to make up for all the missed anniversaries and other occasions. I don't think anyone will contact the psychologist or the neurologist just because I fell down on that score. But when my grandmother started missing birthdays, and then sending two or three cards in a row on the wrong month, we all realised that there was a dramatic change. On its own, not enough to draw conclusions, but enough to draw family attention to other signs of change, which were soon noted and reported.

In her case, this occurred in her early 70's, and was attributed to a treatable cause. The problems ceased and she lived another

20 years or maybe more without more than a level of forgetfulness you might be happy to accept when you are over 90.

So, a lot of assessing and sorting out of problems can often occur without the suggestion of a scan cropping up. A physical examination might reveal more. Signs of stroke could become apparent as could other health conditions that might contribute to dementia or might co-exist such as heart disease or kidney problems. A doctor might order a blood sugar level test, or a thyroid test to check for an under active thyroid. A review of medication might help to find out whether the problems are a side effect of a drug.

If there are still effects that have not been explained by the process so far, neurological examinations such as tests of balance and reflexes and sensory tests might be carried out and these might contribute towards a diagnosis. There are also specific neuropsychological tests for memory and problem-solving, language, maths and spatial ability that are helpful in pinning down changes in suspected dementia.

The reason for getting the diagnosis right and as early as possible is that although if there is a degenerative neurological diagnosis to be made, currently there will be no cure to offer; that is not the same as saying there is no effective treatment. Many interventions, therapies and support measures can help to reduce the impact of the condition on a person's quality of life and improve ability to carry out activities of living, as well as make life a little easier for carers. We have seen in earlier sections that some medications for example that are effective for many people with a particular dementia diagnosis, can seriously exacerbate symptoms in another form of diagnosis.

Also, being clearer about the diagnosis means being able to make a better forecast regarding how the condition is likely to progress, and what help and support might be needed in the future. This can help families to begin to plan ahead. It can take some of the shocks and surprises in the situations ahead, and can allow a measured, thoughtful approach to living accommodation adaptations and other changes and arrangements that might be necessary, rather than rapid reactions to unforeseen crises.

A scan might be recommended at this point for this reason and other potential benefits of having a scan are mentioned further below. In answer to the question heading up this section, 'Should we agree to a scan?' I would say that if my relative was presented with the cognitive problems that we have been discussing, and doctors had explored the other possible reasons as we have just discussed, and now recommended a scan, I would want to encourage my relative to go ahead. I would try to point out that it's like having a photo taken—painless and non-invasive. That of course, doesn't mean the person will cease to be anxious if they do tend to worry about such things. It's the whole procedure of course, and what some people call 'white coat syndrome' or fear of doctors, hospitals and all that goes with it. Also of course, there can be the fear that the scan might confirm an awful diagnosis.

But I have to say that if the anxiety is too great, it's worth backing off and not pushing the point. I might just leave it between the patient and doctor. The thing is, there are limits to the value of the scan in diagnosing dementia. It could of course identify or rule out problems such as a stroke or a tumour. But the doctor would suspect this from the clinical examinations already. But also it can show deviations from normal gross brain anatomy. When we discussed the structure of the brain we talked about the outer part, the cortex being wrinkled with folds and crevices, fairly tightly packed within the skull. There are small cavities or 'ventricles' filled with the cerebrospinal fluid that bathes the brain and spinal cord. A scan could show if the folds of the cortex were less tightly packed and if the ventricles were larger than in a normal brain, meaning that so many cells in the cortex were dying off, and that the brain was visually less dense.

It could also show if there are problems with blood vessels, that is, a stroke or multi infarct dementia (a series of mini strokes) as described earlier. But again, if this is the case, it should already be suspected from the clinical history in which case a scan is important for confirmation.

But without those suspicions a scan in the diagnosis of the type of dementia is not crucial, and would not be definitive, but part of a bigger picture along with all the other information gathered so far. A normal CT scan for example does not rule out dementia.

The most commonly used scan and the type that is most often used to investigate the brains of people with suspected dementia is called a computerised tomography scan, or 'CT' scan, or is sometimes called a CAT scan (computerised Axial Tomography). X-ray equipment and computer software produce black, white and grey pictures of the inside of the body; in this case the brain. The ring-shaped scanner circles around you, taking cross-sectional pictures or 'slices' of your brain. The computer is able to combine the slices and create a 3D picture.

Normally the person will be given an out-patient appointment for the CT scan, and this should take a maximum of half an hour. I would regard it as important to accompany my relative, as a lot of people do find the procedure disturbing. If too anxious and agitated, it should feel okay to the person to change his or her mind about continuing, and go home. If the doctor does feel the scan is very necessary, a sedative can be offered to an anxious patient. I would encourage my relative in this case as the doctor would only say the scan was important with good reason.

The patient might be given an injection that contains a harmless dye, to show up the brain very clearly. The person is asked to lie on a narrow bed, with his or her head near the scanner entrance. A radiographer operates the scanner from an adjacent room, keeping an eye on the patient through a window. The bed moves into the scanner as the pictures are taken. Afterwards the patient can go straight home, unless having been sedated, he or she will have to wait for the okay signal to be given after the effects wear off. Results can't be given at that the time. The pictures need to be analysed and the doctor will arrange for an appointment soon afterwards to discuss and explain what the pictures show, and what they mean.

Less commonly an MRI scan (Magnetic Resonance Imaging) is advised. This results in much higher resolution pictures and is more sensitive to picking up vascular lesions (strokes or ministrokes) than a CT scan is. But the procedure is longer, quite noisy and the sensation can be more claustrophobic. It is a very useful tool though in identifying vascular dementia, and seeing detailed atrophy (cell loss) in specific brain areas even quite early on in the process of dementia.

CT and MRI scans are known as 'structural imaging'. They provide pictures that show the structure of the brain (of course, they can be used to picture any other part of the body. As the name suggests, MRI scans involve passing through a powerful magnet, and therefore there are some circumstances that exclude the people from being considered for this option. No one who has a pacemaker or implants of some kinds or clips to repair an aneurism in a blood vessel at the base of the brain in the past (to resolve a subarachnoid haemorrhage) or any possible metal fragments in the body (for example, a previous metallic splinter in the eye) can be considered for MRI imaging. The process is avoided in the first trimester of pregnancy, and as mentioned, it can be too traumatic for some anxious patients. Obese patients maybe too large to fit into the machine. CT scanning is also avoided in pregnancy due to the X-rays.

Apart from structural imaging, there are other scans that can help to examine the way the brain functions. Currently they are not commonly used to help with diagnosis but in the future could become useful in determining early dementia. Functional imaging is useful in research. Functional MRI (or fMRI) can measure changes in metabolism within the brain. 'Single Photon-Emission Computed Tomography' (SPECT) can make it possible to observe blood distribution in the brain, which is increased in areas that are more active. Positon Emission Tomography (PET) scans show changes in the way glucose and oxygen are metabolized. Where there is cell loss in dementia this activity will be markedly decreased and shows changes in the flow of blood around the brain, giving a good picture of any abnormalities in the functioning of the brain.

Magnetoencephalography (MEG) (you can see why the abbreviations tend to be used) picks up the electromagnetic fields that result from the activity of brain cells.

By comparing functional images taken at certain time intervals in the process of dementia, more can be learned about how the conditions responsible develop, and the effects of new therapies can be observed. This raises the question of whether a person with cognitive problems should choose to accept taking part in research involving brain scanning if invited. This is a very personal and individual decision. It can, for some, be comforting to feel that despite having the misfortune of a particularly unpleasant diagnosis, they can play an important role in research towards developing effective treatments so that future generations maybe spared from these conditions. For others it may add to the distress.

Researchers planning studies have to undergo a rigorous process to obtain ethical approval and this involves demonstrating that their proposed project is likely to be useful, and that any distress caused will be minimal compared to the potential benefits. They also have to show that people taking part will be able to withdraw at any time, and that whether or not they decide to be involved will not affect how they are treated outside of the study.

If a person does decide to take part in research, the purpose of the study and all that the person will undergo has to be explained fully, as far as is possible. Normally the individual must give informed consent before being enrolled. But sometimes researchers maybe able to provide a good reason for wanting to study people with fairly advanced dementia, perhaps to find out if a drug is effective in improving their condition, and it may not be possible to get informed consent as the person may not be capable of understanding the project or making a decision about whether they want to be involved. In this case, after demonstrating to a research ethics committee the importance of the project, and the limited potential for the participant's distress being heavily outweighed by potential benefits of the study, a 'consultee' might be appointed who is often a family carer. This person will help to confirm whether the person is indicating a willingness to take part, despite their lack of ability to give informed consent.

Let us consider scanning for another condition—Multiple sclerosis. This diagnosis is often not an easy one to be sure of when signs and symptoms begin to present. There can be many reasons for the typical neurological symptoms that are associated with MS, and often when these are mild, they can resolve themselves. If symptoms are severe of course, a family physician will refer their patient to a neurologist but if not, often the decision will be to wait and see. Even if a spell of symptoms is mild, if there is a further episode, or a 'relapse' a referral to the neurologist will be made. If the neurologist suspects MS, he or she will initiate a number of tests. These are briefly referred to in the section on Multiple Sclerosis under the heading of 'diagnosis'.

You may have been more concerned in this instance regarding the mention of a Lumbar Puncture than an MRI scan. After checking for any abnormality in the movement ability or sensation and the reflexes, a neurological examination will test for coordination of limbs, eye movements speech and balance. Another test measures how long it takes for signals to the brain after hearing or sight are stimulated. These signals will be slower if the myelin 'sheath' around the axons of neurone in the pathway being tested is disrupted as a result of MS. The procedure is non-invasive, and so doesn't cause any physical discomfort but does involve having small electrodes on the head. It is called an 'electroencephalograph' or more commonly, an 'EEG' There are three main types of 'evoked potential tests' carried out using EEG in the diagnosis of MS. The tests related to hearing (brainstem auditory evoked potentials or 'BAEP') involve listening to a series of clicks through headphones. Visual tests (VEP or visual evoked potentials) involve looking at patterns on a screen. And sensory evoked potential (SEP) involve mild electric shocks given to the limbs.

The Lumbar Puncture, sometimes known as a 'spinal tap' can sound like a more unpleasant prospect. However, it is not carried out these days as often as in the past, only being used when the other tests and examinations are inconclusive. In MS, there are often antibodies in the cerebrospinal fluid, and so the procedure involves drawing some of the fluid from around the spinal cord with a needle, under a local anaesthetic. For this, patients lie on their side, and the needle is inserted into the small of the back, into the space around the cord. From the testimony of people I have accompanied while they have this procedure carried out, the thought of it and the anticipation are much worse than the event, although for some, it can leave a headache. This can last anything from an hour or two, to over a day. But the risk of this occurring is greatly reduced if the patient continues to lie flat for a few hours after the procedure. It has been reported as a more persistent problem by some, and if this were to happen, the neurologist should be consulted to advise on management.

Regarding the scan, and the question of whether to have it, yes, if the neurologist reaches the conclusion following the clinical history-taking, examination and tests, that an MRI scan, as explained above, is to be advised, then it is best regarded as the next necessary step in trying to identify the cause of the symptoms. A 'dye' or rather a 'contrast medium' is usually injected to help highlight inflammation where patches of disrupted myelin occur. It is widely regarded as very accurate in pinpointing lesions, where the myelin is disrupted in the brain or spinal cord in MS. It is reported as being able to confirm a diagnosis in around 90% of people who have MS. However, it does mean that for a minority, the MRI will not be able to show any abnormality even though they do have MS. That is known as a false negative result. Also, sometimes normal aging can lead to some lesions shown on an MRI scan when the person in fact does not have MS. That is called a false positive result.

Clearly MS is a difficult diagnosis to make. All of this uncertainty while different tests go on over time can be very unsettling for patients, and some begin to wonder if 'the experts' really know what they are doing. The reason that the diagnosis is so problematic is because there are such a wide range of symptoms that can be attributed to MS and in each person these symptoms can present individually. Many of these symptoms can occur in other neurological disorders, and some of them can occur occasionally, as an anomaly, in healthy people. There is no single definitive test like a blood test currently that can confirm the condition- diagnosis is achieved by piecing together the various parts of the whole picture. Often the symptoms reported are vague, such as being fatigued, or experiencing sexual dysfunction. These can often be put down to stress. And the symptoms don't tend to remain consistently. Patients describe something strange that they've experienced which didn't persist.

And so, difficult and frustrating though the whole process is bound to be, do trust and bear with your neurologist. It can seem a strange thing to people with no experience of the condition that for many, by the time a firm diagnosis is made, there can be a sense of relief, rather than devastation, in that, 'at last, we all know why I'm having all these problems'.

CT and MRI scans cannot currently identify the changes in the brain related to Parkinson's disease, but they can still be helpful in the process of diagnosis, because of their ability to rule out other potentially confounding causes for neurological problems such as a stroke or a tumour, as we have seen already. Refined MRI scans are being developed that maybe able to clearly detect Parkinson's in future. PET scans can show abnormalities in dopamine cells in the substantia nigra brain area though, and so can be helpful, in distinguishing PD from other movement disorder's causes. Many people who have PD would show an abnormal PET scan, but for some, it maybe inconclusive. For many, the invasiveness and expense and uncertainty with PET scanning in PD, make it a non-appealing option in many cases. As has been the theme throughout this section on scans, it is important to trust the neurologist's clinical judgement, and go with what is recommended, would be my conclusion. We have to accept that the decisions are not always 'cut and dried' and therefore, we do rely on what the neurologist has learned through clinical experience over the years.

Should We Agree to the Medication?

One of the important factors to take on board regarding medication for neurological disorders is that they are prescribed on an individual basis, after consultations and agreement between the person and the professional. What might be the right answer or a prescription worth trying for a particular person in a certain set of circumstances, maybe very wrong for another person even if they share the same diagnosis. I start with this point because so many people do seem to think they're being cheated when they find out that another person has the same diagnosis and is being prescribed different medicine.

The internet can be both fabulously useful, and a problem with regard to this, because at the click of a button you can often find what seem to be clear, simple and obvious answers to your problems, while the neurologist, taking time, may indeed go up a few blind alleys to treat difficult problems but with a systematic approach and in liaison with the patient, or trusted family members if appropriate, will identify the right treatment. So, do ask questions, and express fears. Make sure you have a good rapport with the consultant him or herself, or at least with a specialist nurse who is an expert in your condition. Discussions about taking medication need to feel comfortable and not rushed. By 'comfortable', I mean you should feel at ease about raising questions and concerns about treatments being recommended. If you have looked at the medications on the internet or in a book about medications, and want to know more about say, risks or side effects mentioned, then it should be fine to point that out.

That is not to say that any doctor, whether a GP or a specialist consultant isn't right to make it clear that they are busy people with a lot of patients to see and think about, and that time is precious. There's no problem about being business-like and reminding patients to stick to the point. Hopefully they will be friendly but not a friend as the relationship is professional. But your appointment is your time, and that is precious to you. There maybe a lot of other patients, but not at the moment. If you sense a level of mutual respect for each other's time, knowledge and experience, it should all go well, and there is a much greater chance that decisions about medication will be right for you, or for the person you care for if this is the situation.

Your doctor or specialist nurse or other health professional who might advise about and/or prescribe drugs is expert and professional, and they will have experience to draw on from dealings over the years of what has gone well and not so well with other patients. You may have read about a super treatment or about problems with an established treatment, but he or she is able to set that information into context, and make decisions about how this applies in your case. If you have read some research that found in favour, say, of a treatment, he or she has the knowledge and ability to critique the research, and for example, think about whether the people who took part in the study were likely to be similar to you. So you have to respect that.

Equally, health professionals must respect your knowledge and experience. You know what your condition is really like and how it affects you (or if you're having to speak up for someone that you care for, you are much nearer to understanding this than your doctor or other health professional is). You are an expert on the lived experience of the condition and on what it is like trying to manage it and deal with problems. You know the lived experience also of any medications that have been tried, and whether they make life better or more difficult. The health professional has to respect all of this about you.

This mutual respect should lead to mutual trust. You should be able to trust that the prescription is best for you, going on the evidence so far. You are prepared that it may turn out not to be best; identifying the right treatment can often be a bit like detective work... step by step ruling out the suspects until you know you've got the right one. It can be tough bearing with the process. Similarly, the prescriber has to be able to trust that you will try the treatment according to the instructions if you say you will, and will report accurately the way that they seem to affect you.

So, based on mutual trust and respect, consultations should be productive. If you don't feel you have this, there needs to be a solution. I do know of some really good consultants who nevertheless, don't really have a great knack of striking up a communicative rapport with some patients. It still works well though because the patients are seen by a specialist nurse who has the skill to liaise between the families and the consultant, clarifying to each what the other's perspective is. These nurses are expert and can prescribe or change prescriptions. However any problems about communicating between families and professionals are resolved, they do need to be aired and acknowledged, because if you get to a situation where you take medication sensing that it is doing harm, but not feeling you can say so; or if the doctor has to consider that you might not be following the instructions faithfully, and therefore the effects are difficult to evaluate properly, then there are going to be potentially serious problems.

Why have I laboured this point, about the relationship and rapport with health professionals, you may wonder. Well, because if you get this right, the answer to the question, 'Should we agree to the medication?' will be 'yes'. That is, if it has been prescribed on the basis of mutual understanding. If you don't know what they are for, well, I have to say, I wouldn't take them, but I wouldn't pretend to... I would say that I'll be happy to do so when I'm clear about the reason for having them.

This of course is difficult though, when there are drugs to help a person who due to their diagnosis, cannot grasp or retain an explanation. You have to appreciate that a physician can be put into a very tricky ethical situation... a little like some of those we discussed in the earlier section. Is it right to talk about his patient with you, who presents yourself as a carer? What about confidentiality? Think about the principles referred to in that section about tricky ethical decisions. A 'needs to know' basis is often how the doctor will deal with it- deciding if you need to know in order to work in the patient's best interests.

And what if it is agreed between the carer and the consultant that some medication is in the best interests of the patient, but the patient who apparently doesn't have the capacity to understand why they need it and so refuses to take it. Can you be devious? Would it be ethical to do what I was taught, when I first worked in a psychiatric hospital (now closed), hiding medication in jam and tea? (Many moons ago!).

There have been reports suggesting that it is not uncommon for nurses and care staff members working in residential care and nursing homes to hide medicines in food and in beverages, notably in Norway and also in South East England. No doubt it is a much more widespread practice than that, and the condition most associated with this practice appears to be dementia. I'm sure family members have resorted to this at home as well. When this is carried out in a formal setting, by paid staff including professionals, it is not generally evident in the records. Studies that have investigated the practice are few and far between but tend to ask staff members in isolation. If mixing the medicine in food is mentioned in patient records, there tends to be no clear explanation of how the decision to do this was reached.

The practice, it seems, tends to be most likely to be adopted when patients are aggressive, or difficult to manage because of poor cognition interfering with their ability to carry out activities of living, or to act compliantly when being assisted to wash, dress, eat, mobilise and so on. And I have to say, I don't find any of this surprising. It's fine to be told that this is wrong. So it is. But I often found as a staff nurse and as a carer that people - some managers and some physicians come to mind- who reminded you that you mustn't do it, and who simultaneously pointed out the importance of the medication were not prepared to demonstrate to how to get the person to comply. That, I feel, creates an environment conducive to secrecy and dishonesty.

Openness is needed. I never hesitated to write down what I had done in the nursing notes, even if I thought it was the wrong thing to do. It forced the issue to the table for discussion and decisions. That's because, while those carrying out an improper practice do it covertly, senior people can ignore it as a problem, knowing they will be able to claim ignorance about the practice if it does ever come to a head. The person actually hiding the medicine can take the wrap. That was no longer an option for managers once I wrote it in the notes and pointed it out to them. They now officially knew what was going on, and had to get involved with sorting out a solution.

And that raised the question—what is the solution? Oh dear, I'm beginning to wish I'd kept this book simple, and avoided so many sticky topics without straight answers. But, well, we're here now. So let's try to decide what's best to do. (Notice I said what's 'best', rather than what's 'right'. You can't always do what's completely right; that's my experience).

The United Kingdom Psychiatric Pharmacy Group (2009) (UKPPG) are fairly clear about their position. A sub-committee was set up especially to consider this problem and the larger group has adopted their recommendations. They acknowledge that it can be necessary to give some people medication in their best interests even if the person is unable to give consent. They say that treatment can be given to a person who won't take it if it is given openly, if it is in the best interests of the person who doesn't have the mental capacity to make their own informed choice. But these 'best interests' can't be trivial. If you are going to save a life or improve the person's condition, or save a deterioration by giving a treatment that is in accordance with standard recognized practice by an appropriate professional body, then you should be able to defend giving the medication, providing you have a good rationale for deciding that the person does not have capacity, as we have discussed earlier.

But it should not happen on the basis of a decision made subjectively by an individual such as a nurse, who just feels it seems a sensible idea. The UKPPG suggest that in the absence of nationally agreed standards or protocols determining when this practice might be appropriate, how to make decisions and how to carry it out, there must be locally agreed procedures. And the health professional or carer concerned must make sure they find out about them and work within them in a culture of openness, so that other professionals are aware of and can monitor and review the situation as changes in circumstances occur.

However, while giving the medication without consent maybe acceptable in these circumstances, the Royal College of Psychiatrists Ethics Sub Committee are clear that the medicine should not be disguised so that the person is not aware that they are taking it. That makes hiding medicine in jam or a flavoured drink an unethical practice that should not be happening. Of course, it might be okay to give medicine in this way if the person does know and by agreement, finds it easier to take when mixed. That would not be covert, but there is another issue to consider here, of whether the method of taking the medicine is compliant with the instructions provided by the pharmacist or manufacturer. For example, some medicines can cause harm if the outer layer is damaged before swallowing, and so they mustn't be halved or crushed; and some must be taken with water in an empty stomach. So these checks must be made with the pharmacy.

In these difficult circumstances then, a local policy should be established and followed openly and should take account of the following general principles.

Hiding medicine in food and drinks covertly without the knowledge of the person receiving the medicine is never acceptable. If the person is refusing medicine, it must not be given in food or drink, regardless of whether the person has capacity or not.

The decision to mix medicines in food and drink with the person's agreement should only happen if certain steps have been taken:

There should be a multi-disciplinary review to establish whether the medication is really important enough to the person's health or quality of life to justify these extreme measures.

If the person wishes to take the medicine in food or drinks because of difficulties in taking it as prescribed normally, then steps should be taken to assess why this is. For example by involving a speech and language therapist if there are swallowing problems, then reasonable efforts must be made to resolve the underlying problem.

If medicine must be given to the person in his or her interests, without consent, there should be multi-disciplinary discussions to establish whether it may have to be carried out under mental health legislation. The law of course differs in different countries but essentially, it is a decision about treating the person in their interests without consent, but as far as is possible with their knowledge and understanding, and never by being devious or deceitful.

If the medicine is to be given in food, the doctor should make the prescription clear regarding how this is to be administered and with what. The pharmacy should be consulted to ensure the administration method is pharmaceutically sound. Medical and nursing notes should openly document the practice that is carried out and all relevant discussions with the multi-disciplinary team, including close relatives caring for a person where applicable.

Often, as this process is entered into, and the various team members begin to contribute their expertise, problems tend to be resolved, often rather simply. Perhaps, the medication is felt not to be so crucial as originally perceived, or difficulties with swallowing are overcome, or a syrup rather than a tablet form of the medicine turns out to be more acceptable to the person. The key point about it all I feel, as you may have become aware, is openness. Don't carry these problems around on your own, or endure the guilt feelings that are bound to go with secrecy. This isn't just your problem to deal with—share it. But equally, don't feel bad about it if up to now you have been crushing and hiding medicine in honey—it's understandable, and you're certainly not alone. Forgive yourself. Get over it and get help to find a better solution, that's all. It's most likely that it is not your fault. You just got caught up in a culture where people didn't question what had become regarded as standard practice.

So, the general point about whether to agree to the medication is to do so on the basis of an individual decision arrived at with a consensus between the consultant or other relevant prescribing health professional, the patient and the carer. One of the main things to consider is whether 'problems' being treated are indeed problems from the perspective of the person taking the medicine. There is a danger that without a good discussion, a health professional could run to the conclusion that the observable signs need to be corrected, as a priority above less measurable effects of the condition, even if the patient does not share this idea of prioritizing. Therefore, a tremor might be treated, or involuntary movement, such as chorea in limbs reduced to the satisfaction of both the carer and the physician, when the person concerned was happy to live with these effects, and is not happy with, for example, a limiting effect that the drugs seem to have on voluntary movement.

What for some might be liberation from a socially stigmatizing problem with involuntary movement, for others it might be a greater problem than the original symptom that the physician sought to remedy. Such misunderstandings can be a huge source of frustrations all round, as the patient feels no one is prepared to consider what he or she needs; the health professional feels that all the efforts to measurably improve the impact of the disorder are received ungratefully; and the carer feels caught between the two, perhaps having to try to defend each point of view to the other person, and only getting a negative response from both directions. What an unfortunate nightmare this can be, and just the kind of scenario that can end up with the patient nodding in agreement at the clinic, despite no intention of adhering to the advice. Then, when there is another problem, and the health professional advises a drug that really would be very helpful, this advice and prescription also might be discarded quietly at home, because of the breakdown with communications.

I reiterate then, the importance of deciding about appropriate medication in open, multi-disciplinary discussions.

How will We Cope Psychologically and Spiritually?

It's a very individual thing, the way people deal with having a degenerative neurological condition; or perhaps being the carer for someone with Parkinson's, Huntington's, Alzheimer's disease or one of the other conditions we have been considering.

Different people attach different meanings to having such a diagnosis, personally, or in the family. For some, it's bad luck. It just happens. For others, there must be a reason... they find themselves asking 'why me?' 'Why now?' And some feel they have at least an inkling about the kinds of reasons that could be at the bottom of it. Often, people feel it's their own fault. They didn't live the right life-style, eating the right things, exercising, didn't read enough mentally challenging books, do puzzles or use 'brain trainers'; or perhaps they think they made a 'wrong choice', living near electric pylons or in a hard water area containing a lot of aluminium, or some other substance that is felt to be unhealthy. (I'm not for a minute suggesting any of these as causes by the way).

Some people feel it's some sort of curse on the family or perhaps a punishment or a trial from God. 'These things are sent to try us', I've heard many people say. Phrases like that role off some people's tongues and it doesn't mean too much. But for others, it is the crux of their belief about these matters.

Should nurses and carers be concerned with spiritual aspects or is it an area beyond our scope?

Since the days of Florence Nightingale spiritual care has been central to nursing. The founder of nursing as an educated profession wrote: 'The needs of the spirit are as critical to health as those individual organs which make up the body'. The 1946 NHS Act identified Hospital Chaplains as an integral part of the new National Health Service, which was born on 5th July, 1948. The World Health Organisation 2005 defines palliative care as: 'An approach that improves the quality of life of patients and their families facing the problems associated with life-threatening illness, through the prevention and relief of suffering by means of early identification and impeccable assessment and treatment of pain and other problems, physical, psychosocial and spiritual'.

Department of Health (UK) documents 'Religion or Belief: A Practical Guide For The NHS' (2009) and 'End Of Life Care Strategy' (2008) stresses the importance of regarding spiritual care as an essential part of health care for people with conditions that threaten life. The latter makes the point: 'Many people need to discover their own way of making sense out of what is happening to them. So allowing the person to express anger, guilt, sadness and reconciliation is an important aspect of caring. It is important that spirituality is part of the assessment process, so that it becomes an integral part of care and is reviewed at each stage of the pathway'.

So frankly, I would say 'yes' we should be concerned with spiritual aspects, and 'no', it is not an area beyond our scope. So, let's consider how people cope, spiritually and emotionally, or psychologically.

Coping

How people begin to make sense of the situation can have a strong bearing on the way they will cope with it, or manage.

There is a lot of theory about coping with health changes. Some of the ideas about how people cope resemble Freudian 'defence mechanisms'. In this view, we may deal with life's stressful circumstances by using strategies such as denial (not consciously accepting that things have changed) and carrying on as though everything was fine. Our conscious mind refuses to accept that it has happened because it is too much to face. Or projection, that is, allowing ourselves to react emotionally, for example angrily, but not facing up to the reality of what the anger is about. So we 'project' the angry feelings on to someone or something else. There are many other examples.

The ideas of Lazarus and Folkman (1984) arose from the view that how we deal with stresses in life such as health changes is more dynamic. It is the result of continuing interaction between cognition—the way we think about, understand and perceive the situation, and our emotions. Most theories before this were either about how we think (cognition); or about emotional responses to situations. But Lazarus and Folkman broke new ground by theorising about the interactions between these two components of our being.

In this concept, when a life event happens, we try to think of how significant it is for our lives and potentially how stressful. Then we assess what reserves we have to be able to deal with it. We then set about coping predominantly using either 'problem-focussed' coping, or 'emotional-focussed coping'. In problem-focussed coping, we take a problem solving approach, trying to address what has happened, reducing or if possible eliminating the impact. But in emotional-focussed coping, we don't deal with the problem, we just try to manage our emotions towards the problem. For some people, turning to alcohol, drugs, or becoming incredibly busy, convincing ourselves we have too many commitments to be able to deal with the problem, can be ways of managing emotions instead of the problem.

Most forms of coping could have the potential to be effective in some circumstances, and can be counter-productive in others. Given a degenerative neurological diagnosis, I don't know how

I'd react. But I have a feeling that initially, going for a few drinks might feature. And after that, I can imagine having a couple more. That's me- I've done it in the past with bad and with good news. I'm not proud, but well, that's how it is.

Please don't knock it for someone like me. I think it helps. Don't be tempted to drive though, if you've been drinking alcohol. Get a cab, and if you can, stop before you're ill. When you begin to feel the bad news isn't so awful, you've probably had enough. For some people, this is entirely the wrong approach. So it's not advice I'm just relating my probable first reaction. I say 'probable', but as I mentioned in the last paragraph, I really have no idea how I might react. And it has to be borne in mind that a lot of people find that by the time there is a diagnosis, it has been obvious for some time that all is not well, and some say the news comes as a relief.

Anyway, if it did happen to me and I did have those drinks, I know that very soon, the strategy would outlive its usefulness, and become counter-productive. I should move into another approach. That can be difficult, if you have found a strategy that brings short term comfort, and saves you facing reality. You need to know that it's a problem if you get stuck in that unproductive response, and problems need to be acknowledged and resolved, with help if necessary.

I mention these ideas about coping only briefly to point out that it can be useful to think about how people we care for and family members might be dealing with their circumstances. We aren't expert in this area, but we can be supportive and understanding, and might alert experts if we are concerned that inappropriate and ineffective strategies are potentially harming the person's well-being.

It can help us to appreciate how some people might deal with living with a degenerative neurological diagnosis, if we think about and try to understand something of the kinds of factors that might influence their response. As well as considering ideas about coping strategies, it can be useful to have some knowledge of the person's previous outlook on life, the meaning of it, and the meaning of ill-health, particularly degenerative neurological disease.

Some Broad Cultural and Religious Attitudes to Illness

What follows is a very brief comment on the attitudes, values and beliefs about these matters, commonly associated with some cultural traditions and religions. It is important to appreciate that it docsn't follow that someone who is a member of or practices a particular religion necessarily looks at life, health or ill-health, the way I might portray as the religious view here. That's because:

1. The presentations here are brief and superficial just to give a flavour of the diversity of approaches that can be considered. The truth about the religious or cultural view will be much more complex, and there is not room here to analyse the complexity.

2. Individuals within a culture or religion don't all share exactly the same views. Faiths have to be interpreted to be lived. Not all who share a faith necessarily share the same interpretation of it, especially regarding how the belief might be applied in different contextual circumstances.

3. Life experiences tend to change how we see things and how we feel about beliefs we may have been sure of previously.

4. Some people who have never really taken a religion they may

have been brought up in seriously, for example, suddenly find they are drawn closer to it and draw comfort from it when face with a degenerative illness.

5. On the other hand, some who have been devoted to a religious belief all their life, react by feeling let down by it and may lose their faith.

6. Some steadfastly hang on to what they have always known.

Whatever their reaction, a supportive, non-judgmental and non-directive listening approach is bound to help the person work out the best way they can handle their condition. Getting to the point where they have worked out their attitude to spiritual and emotional aspects of the diagnosis in many cases will involve periods of uncertainty and contradictions. It's good to allow these twists and turns without trying to tell the person what is right.

Please regard these following brief comments on some; just a few of the many cultural traditions and religions as aids towards appreciating a wide range of possible views, values and beliefs. For professional carers and nurses particularly, never fall into the trap of telling someone what you think they ought to think because of their faith. Be a listener, and allow space for the person to think through their attitude to their condition, and whether it has changed or is changing. Respect their view, whether or not it is static currently or changing. The following are only examples of positions within faiths or cultural backgrounds. These comments do not attempt to explain or give some sort of overview or the account of the tradition.

They focus only on attitudes to illness such as a neurodegenerative disease. There are many other equally important traditions of course. There is no attempt to address all perspectives here. Just to consider a small range of views to help to foster an appreciation for the diversity of attitudes we may need to support, when caring for people with neurological disease.

Atheism

Within this very broad term there are a multitude of values and beliefs about life, its meaning and the significance of and reasons for health problems such as neurological disease. Nurses and carers, particularly those who have a deep religious conviction need to understand and respect that '...'atheism', does not mean (as is often assumed among many religious people) an absence of any belief. Instead, the position held by an individual who would describe him or herself as an atheist is often as deeply rooted in thought and experience, and handed on values as is any other faith system. Of course, someone who has never given much thought about why we are here, and whether life or illness have meaning might also describe him or herself as atheist.

So, there are many possible positions, as there are within all beliefs. Some people find peace and comfort in atheism, where, with no god to contend with, they can embrace their illness that will lead to death, without having to contend with ideas of after-life, and continued strife to atone for an imperfect earthly existence. There are many ways of looking at living on though, within a 'no god' position. Would I exist as a person, if there was no representation of me in another person's mind? What makes me who I am, is how I am perceived in other people's heads. When I die, those perceptions and representations, memories will remain and be passed on. Many people with children and grandchildren see their lives as continuing through their inherited genes... a little of me in my offspring, living on.

Others feel that if they do something while alive, that has a lasting impact, they live on in this way. Artists such as Van Gough, musicians such as John Lennon, and reformers such as Wilberforce or Martin Luther King are often thought to be living on in the sense that the world remains a better place because of their lasting impact. We don't have to be so publicly appreciated to leave behind a living legacy. We have touched more lives than we will ever know.

These are just some of many ways that an eventually terminal condition such as a degenerative neurological disease can be embraced by a person who describes him or herself as an atheist. There must be many more ways.

While long term illness such as degenerative neurological disorder can be come to terms with, and accepted, a faith in logical science gives us some control over events. We are not at the mercy of a power that decides whether to answer prayers and give us health. Therefore, it is within our capacity over time to defeat these conditions.

Buddhism

Buddha lived in India almost 2,600 years ago. The first of his four noble teachings was that life is 'Dukkha'. This word has no exact English translation. It has three aspects. The first is suffering or pain. This may include physical pain, mental anguish and emotional pain. The second aspect of 'Dukkha' is impermanence. This includes happiness, success and even spiritual bliss, anything that is only temporary. The third aspect is 'conditioned states'. According to Buddha we and everything are all conditioned, that is, affected by something or someone else.

What we call 'I', or the 'self', in Buddhism is only a convenient label for an impermanent group of attributes, that will not be the same in any two consecutive moments. So, the world is holistic, and separate entities such as 'I', 'myself' don't really make good sense in a view where everything acts on everything else.

Health in Buddhism is much more than an absence of disease. It is holism. It can be positively or negatively affected by 'kamma'.

Illness may have its origin in kamma from the past. This does not mean a belief in fate then. Relief of suffering and a cure should be sought. Anyway, there maybe a physical cause. There is a responsibility for personal health that is, living an unhealthy lifestyle may result in illness. The responsibility is shared by society. Health is harmony between mind and body, which are not separate. Harmony is to be strived for but is not attainable at all times and therefore, illness, including a degenerative neurological disorder that will result in death, is inevitable given our fragile condition.

Working to relieve the suffering of those who are diagnosed with such a condition, and assisting them to achieve harmony as far as possible contributes towards good kamma.

Christianity

Christians are so called because they are 'followers of Christ'. Within Christianity, there are many denominations. For example, the Roman Catholic church, Greek and Russian Orthodox churches, the Anglican, Methodist and Baptist churches. There are many more, and within these churches, there are various distinct communities. So, beliefs within Christianity are very diverse. And so are attitudes towards a diagnosis of say Alzheimer's disease, Parkinson's disease or a stroke.

With regard to suffering and illness, Christ who was God made man, lived and died 2000 years ago. He was cruelly tormented and killed on a cross. The image of the suffering Christ is a reminder that suffering can have a purpose and can be healing: a part of the salvation of souls, in reparation for the sins of the world.

That is not to say that suffering isn't to be avoided. Note, it can play a part in healing souls, uniting Christians with Christ. But it is not good in itself and the relief of suffering is the responsibility of all Christians. The belief that there can be good in accepting the unavoidable consequences of a neurological disorder as in a way, sharing the weight of Christ's cross, doesn't mean that Christians don't become shocked, depressed and so on at the news, like anyone else. This belief doesn't protect them from those reactions, but it can help some Christians to work through them.

Christians who have spells of losing their faith during suffering, take heart in the words of Christ from the cross, before dying: 'My God, my God, why have you forsaken me?'

Hinduism

In Hinduism, suffering is regarded as an inevitable consequence of negative actions either in this life or a past life. It is not a punishment, just a natural result. Unlike in Judaism, where there is no point in asking 'why me' or 'why now', in Hinduism, these are relevant questions. It may not be possible to work out exactly what the reason is, but the answer would be that the individual can be reassured that these are the right circumstances at the right time. If it doesn't seem fair, the person can be assured that it is okay to feel that way, but debts accrued from past actions are being settled.

Pain and suffering in the body will not harm the soul, and by way of offering comfort, the person is reminded that the pain (living with a neurological disorder in this case) is only a temporary situation. Attachment to the world is seen as an obstacle on the path towards God (Brahman) and Hindus seek detachment in which no earthly pain can cause suffering. Hindus can learn how to detach from pain whether emotional and physical.

The answers to problems about suffering need to come from a person who shares the Hindu faith. It is not appropriate to give that advice as a nurse or carer who, like myself, is not a Hindu. But we can listen and ask, 'How have you learned to deal with painful situations in the past? How well has this worked for you? Do you feel you can try this now, in relation to living with your diagnosis of a neurological condition?'

Islam

Islam shares with Christianity the belief that after this life on earth, there is another life with a transformed body. Depending on how we have lived we will live the afterlife in paradise or hell, after the day of judgment. That said, as with Christians also, there is a wide variety of interpretation among individuals, with some regarding these teachings as largely symbolic, and others understanding them in literal terms. Also, many who describe themselves as 'Muslim' and who regard this as integral to their being, do not practice the faith in the sense of attending a mosque or saying daily prayers.

Seeking medical treatment in illness and taking a responsible attitude to health is important in Islam, but in the absence of recovery, disease is accepted with patience and prayers. Death is seen as a journey towards God, and so should not be feared or resented. This can help in coming to terms with a long term neurological, degenerative disease, but doesn't make the acceptance easy. All individuals are prone to despair depression and anxiety, and all can feel emotional as well as physical pain. Faith gives us goals to aspire to. It doesn't prevent us from going through these aspects of the human experience.

Giving time to allow someone to vocalize how they are grappling with their beliefs and struggling to draw strength from them to deal with their predicament, is helpful. Pointing out how they are 'supposed' to view the situation is unhelpful.

Judaism

The appropriate response for Jews towards any human tragedy and suffering is comfort and consolation. The story of Job, who was plagued by a long series of devastating misfortunes illustrates the sheer futility of asking God 'why?' The reasons are beyond us. There is a common opinion an acceptance that to ask 'why' is natural, but the duty of comforters is to help the person come to terms with the challenge posed by the tragic circumstances. In this case, living with a degenerative neurological disorder. The challenge of life is to rise above disasters and teach and contribute to the building of the 'new Jerusalem'. Grieving is acceptable and encouraged, but for a limited time. After that, a person should not wallow in their sorrows. This is a waste of time when there is too much 'building' left do. This refers to the building of goodness and morality. In good time when the building is complete, Jews believe that they will be comforted.

As indicated with regard to the other faiths listed above, there are wide differences in the way that individuals interpret teachings, and in taking on the role of comforter, a good listener is needed. It may not be clear to the individual how to apply these general principles in the current and personal circumstances. It may take time to think it all through and a carer or nurse should not assume that it will be easy or even possible to relate the teachings to their own situation. Just being there, supportive and non-judgemnental will help this process.

Sikhism

A 'Sikh' is a 'disciple' of the one, timeless, universal God of all of humanity. For Sikhs, the body perishes eventually, but the soul is immortal. The soul is part of God, and it yearns for reunion with God.

For Sikhs, suffering is not caused by God, but God allows it to happen, as it tests courage and faith. It also has the effect of drawing out good from others in the society who show compassion and work to heal and ease the suffering. Sikhs are taught not to fear death as it is not the end of life. The soul lives on after death and is reincarnated. A person maybe reborn frequently as a human or as an animal.

There is only a chance to end the cycle of rebirth because only humans, not animals can distinguish between right and wrong. And it is good behaviour that can free a person from the cycle.

When Sikhs are ill, prayers are said and hymns sung, to ask for God's help and for peace. It is important to make the effort to get well and to accept medical intervention, including pain relief. But comfort in the acceptance of a degenerative neurological disorder will come from the understanding of this suffering as the path to God and the release from the cycle of reincarnation.

There are many more of these broad perspectives. As has been emphasized, people who identify with them, never the less have their own personal perspectives. And that tends to change with life experience, particularly in the wake of acquiring a life altering diagnosis. An open, flexible approach to understanding how individuals endeavour to come to grips with living with a neurological disorder, and a warm, listening ear will be much more appreciated than an account of your own perspective on how to deal with it. That can be difficult if you do have fairly strong views. But if you can, it is worth putting them aside and allowing space for the person's efforts to do his or her own working out.

For formal carers and nursing staff, this is essential. Would you be prepared to pray along with the person, or join in hymns, attend services, regardless of whether these seemed to fit with your own practices? It's worth considering what level of support you maybe happy to give, before it becomes an issue, so that you can have a considered response ready. Whatever the answer, early on, find out whom to contact to enable the person to practice their faith as they wish. Find out what they would require to happen in the event of death. Check that this is all documented with step by step instructions. Imagine the situation occurring, say in a nursing home, at night, with a temporary nurse on duty, and make the instructions easy for that person to follow. Always plan for the most difficult scenario– if that is covered, everyone ought to be able to cope. Now and then check if team members know what to do. Someone who kindly read a draft of the above section asked me 'where do you stand then, with regard to these beliefs?' I think perhaps the response should be 'I am a nurse. When you are faced with coming to terms with a diagnosis and its consequences, I'll stand by you'.

Can Complementary Therapies be Helpful?

I have encountered many people in the course of my nursing career who have conditions such as Insulin Dependent Diabetes Mellitus (IDDM), or Asthma, for example. I don't think anyone would consider swapping the main medical treatment they are prescribed for a complementary or 'alternative' medicine. They might use these for related purposes, perhaps to reduce anxiety for example or help sleep, but not, I'm sure as the treatment. That's because people with IDDM know that their insulin, taken as prescribed, works. People with asthma tend to trust their inhalers equally well again, because they work. As a general rule, if you can ask a lot of people what the treatment is for a condition, and you get the same answer repeatedly, you know that the treatment is effective pretty much across the board. But if you get a wide range of responses, you generally can safely conclude that none of the treatments are effective for everyone with the condition.

Take headache for example; ask people what works for them. Some will say aspirin, some paracetamol and others ibruprofen. And that's just those who give 'mainstream'– you might say western– pharmaceutical answers. Some will say they lie down in a dark room with a cool flannel over their heads while others will say they drink a lot of water. My friend insists having a couple of beers works for him, even though it doesn't make any sense to me as I think that should surely make the problem worse. But I have been with him when he's complained of a thumping head, and we have gone to the pub. After his couple of pints, he seems fine. This is someone who rarely takes alcohol otherwise! Well, you have to take the person's word for it, you can't measure a headache in the way you could measure insulin levels for people with diabetes, or respiratory output for a person with asthma, and objectively demonstrate the change that the treatment has brought about.

What about back pain? Some swear by acupuncture, some visit the chiropractor; the osteopath, physiotherapist and some feel nothing will work until they have surgery. Again, none of these approaches are effective for everybody and people often turn to one expert and then another until they find someone they feel is doing them some good.

Well, the reason that the use of 'complementary' and 'alternative' medicine often collectively referred to as 'CAM' is so widespread among people with a degenerative neurological diagnosis is that conditions are currently without any cure, and are all associated with diverse symptoms, specific to individuals, for which there is no 'catch all' medical solution. In most cultures now, I feel, there does seem to be an increasing expectation that for every diagnosis, there should be some effective treatment available. We no longer seem so prepared as perhaps many have been in the past, to just accept all the anguish and suffering that seem to inevitably accompany ill-health. I am sure that this is a very positive aspect of our human condition, motivating us to take control, and feel responsible for tackling the challenges we come up against, rather than writing situations off as hopeless unless from an external source we are handed a miracle. This can work well for people for whom there is no god and are no miracles, and can equally work will, for people who experience their God working within them and inspiring them and for whom the power of their God's miracles is internalised.

And the result of so many people being unprepared to accept that there isn't a treatment or intervention to turn to that will at least control or reduce the symptoms, if not eliminate them, is phenomenal growth in complementary or alternative medicine. But, 'alternative' to what? You might say, probably correctly, 'to mainstream medicine'. And of course, this is all relative.

What might be considered 'mainstream' practice or treatment in one culture may well be unconventional in another. So as people from all cultures become more prepared to look for something to turn to from outside of their traditional scope, we experience a great deal of overlap. Some folk who have come from a line of generations reliant solely on herbal preparations or tribal rituals are happy to branch out into western pharmaceutical drugs, while people who have grown up under the umbrella of a 'science-based' western health service and have traditionally regarded 'primitive' approaches as suspicious, or perhaps 'quaint' but groundless, are more inclined to try these approaches.

We have mentioned pharmacological treatments along the way, so let's briefly consider other therapies, and how they might be helpful for some people with some of the neurological diagnoses we have discussed. For simplicity, despite my acknowledgement above that what might be considered 'alternative' or 'complementary' to one person could be 'conventional' to another, I hope it's acceptable to you, that I will just refer to all the interventions that aren't pharmaceutical, discussed below as 'complementary'. A couple of points about complementary therapies that are making them increasingly popular are the fact that on the whole, people tend to regard them as safe, and without unwanted side effects like those often associated with drugs. And while drugs for the most part target specific symptoms complementary therapies characteristically treat the whole person. This is known as a 'holistic' approach.

The term 'complementary' is fitting I think because as a nurse, I feel I must strongly advocate that you seek orthodox advice first, and work with your GP, consultant / or specialist nurse and other health professionals with regulated qualifications before trying these approaches, regardless of reports about them by friends, family or internet sites. Reach concordance with the professionals and discuss any complementary approaches you are considering, to check. There is no problem about having both treatments. The pleasant perception I mentioned that people have, about the safety of complementary medicine in general isn't necessarily justified in every case. Some of them can be harmful in certain circumstances, especially in conjunction with some drugs. The way drugs work can be altered by some herbal treatments or other substances.

Acupuncture

One of the criticisms generally about complementary therapies is that there hasn't been enough hard evidence to help substantiate claims that are made about their effectiveness. Lee et al (2008) reviewed all the randomised controlled trials, that is, rigorous experimental studies where some people are given a treatment, in this case acupuncture, and are compared to groups of similar people given no treatment or a placebo, to identify any apparent effect of the treatment, that they found in a systematic search. A placebo is a 'sham' medical intervention. Placebos can have an effect perhaps because the psychological experience of being 'treated' is healing to some extent for some people. There is a fairly common belief that the reason some people find complementary therapies effective is because of this placebo effect. They believe it will work, and they feel better; a matter of faith maybe, rather than any power in the treatment itself. So this study by Lee et al sought to establish by looking at a large number of these trials, whether acupuncture is more effective than no treatment at all, or 'treatment' with a placebo.

They concluded that the evidence in favour of the effectiveness of acupuncture for Parkinson's disease was 'unconvincing'. It doesn't mean that they found acupuncture to be ineffective. It means that the studies were not of a good enough quality to be able to aid any decision about whether acupuncture is effective for PD. A typical problem was that they didn't have very many people in each group in the study, and so if a few people began to improve after acupuncture, it could have easily happened just by coincidence. Lee et al call for more and better quality research studies to address this question. I mention this because the picture is pretty similar currently regarding complementary therapies generally; there just is not enough sound evidence one way or the other. One reason maybe that researchers interested in investigating complementary therapies don't manage to attract funding to do so from governments or large businesses in the way that people carrying out drug trials do.

Whatever the reason for all this, for the time being, we do tend to have to generally rely on our beliefs about these things, what people tell us about their experiences, and then our own experiences if we try them. A little later in this chapter, I'm going to re-visit this notion that experimental trials as described above are the way to establish how effective complementary therapies can be. Many people would say, 'Who cares how it works?' Psychologically, biologically or in whatever way if it helps, and as long as the doctor agrees there is no harm, it's worth sticking with it. One thing about complementary therapists is they usually have a lot more time to spare with their patients than doctors do, and perhaps that factor in itself is therapeutic.

But for many other people there is no need to be sceptical about a therapy such as acupuncture which has helped alleviate many ailments for millions of people since ancient times. Acupuncture involves inserting very fine, thread-like needles into particular points in the body and manipulating them skillfully. It is a conventional treatment in Chinese traditional medicine. The acupuncture points in the body run along 'meridian' lines. But Classical Chinese acupuncture is not the only type; there is also Japanese, Tibetan, Korean and Vietnamese acupuncture practiced throughout the world. The fact that acupuncture has been found effective for many conditions in many cultures since ancient times and that this continues to be the case is acknowledged by a World Health Organisation review (WHO 2003). But they conclude that only national health authorities can determine the diseases, symptoms and conditions for which acupuncture treatment can be recommended'.

In Chinese traditional medicine there is a concept of 'liver blood', taking nourishment to muscles tendons and bones, and when the 'liver blood' is deficient and unable to do this work effectively, a condition known as 'liver wind' can arise, causing problems with movement such as those seen in Parkinson's. These concepts do not exist in western medicine. By locating the needles at points in the body that relate to liver wind, and sometimes also treating with Chinese herbs, therapists claim that symptoms of Parkinson's can be reduced and in some cases the progress of the disease can be halted.

Acupuncturists explain Multiple Sclerosis in four stages. A stage with no current symptoms, although there may have been symptoms previously is considered to be one, a stage where there are symptoms but these are often sudden and are 'superficial' in that the MS disease hasn't pervaded the body deeply is stage two. Stages three and four are where there is deeper disease associated with progressive symptoms. The aim of acupuncture is to hold MS in stage one as far as possible and for as long as possible.

Acupuncture is claimed by some to be able to increase verbal skills, motor ability, cognitive function and lift the mood in people with Alzheimer's disease. More general benefits associated with neurological conditions that are claimed frequently and are not necessarily specific to diagnosis include improvements in depression and anxiety, dizziness, sleep problems and problems with urinary and kidney function, headaches, pain and eye problems.

So acupuncture maybe helpful to many people, and certainly if people find it effective in easing ways in which their neurological condition has impacted on them, when other interventions have failed to help, they are of course likely to stay with it.

The relationship with the therapist and his or her experience, knowledge and skill are bound to be important factors in whether the treatment is effective or not. Of course, acupuncture is an invasive treatment, and so administered inappropriately may have the potential to harm. Countries vary in the way that acupuncture is regulated. In the United States specialised practitioners are known as 'Licensed Acupuncturists', or LAc's, and each state stipulates how much training they must undergo to maintain registration. Similarly other health professionals such as physicians, podiatrists and so on who additionally practice acupuncture also must undertake minimum training and these and Lac's must update regularly in order to keep practising.

Canadian law in British Columbia and in Ontario regulate the profession and in Australia states vary with Victoria alone maintaining an operational registration board. Some states have 'skin penetration' legislation that covers acupuncture, and can be used to uphold standards.

In China only doctors can perform acupuncture as this is part of their mainstream medicine. But in many countries acupuncture is not regulated as a profession, although legislation such as that to do with 'assault' maybe relevant if there are claims of improper practice. In Britain for example, there is no specific legal regulation. This does mean that anyone can set up as an acupuncturist and begin practising without training. An impressive web site and a brass plate on the door can help to create an image of professionalism. But many become voluntary members of acupuncture organisations that set and maintain their own standards and codes of practice. Examples are the British Acupuncture Council; the British Medical Acupuncture Society; the Acupuncture Association of Chartered Physiotherapists and the British Academy of Western Acupuncture.

In countries without legal regulation, it is advisable to check that practitioners- not only of acupuncture, but of any therapy or intervention regarded in that country as 'alternative' or 'complementary', do belong to an established, well-reputed self-regulatory body that insists on members maintaining specified levels of training, and standards of practice.

Alexander Technique

Sadly, I just missed the possibility of bumping into Frederick Alexander. Like Albert Einstein, he died in the year I was born (1955). He (Alexander) apparently had experienced vocal problems and developed a way of training his muscles, by recognising and releasing tension in them to solve his condition. He then taught the method widely, to address many conditions related to muscular control. Of course many of the problems caused by the degenerative neurological disorders we have discussed are brought about because of the loss of effective communication between the nervous system and muscles. You may have noticed that I gave my age away there, and another personal admission is that I would never have chosen to go into nursing, as I wanted to be a singer. But I really don't sing very well; I wonder if I had been able to meet Alexander, he could have fixed that. Nursing has turned out a fabulous choice however. I digress, sorry.

Particularly with the Alexander technique, there is a focus on posture, balance and alignment of the skull and vertebrae down the spine. The technique is often taught on a one-to-one basis between the patient or client and the expert. The technique is famous for helping people to improve confidence and overcome stress, and of course, to train the voice. Muscular pain apparently responds well. During nursing training, our class was visited by a teacher of the Alexander technique, and I had never complained about back ache that I found problematic from time to time, because at the time I felt that admitting that might jeopardise my job prospects. Some nurses were prepared to tolerate a male nurse in the ward despite the perceived lack of competence with many of the female skills, provided the man looked as though he could do a lot of the heavy lifting. Things have changed of course, there is supposed to be no lifting and only 'manual handling', and the traditional view of separate male/female skills seems to have eased off.

But anyway, the Alexander technique teacher saw through me easily and pointed out exactly where I experience pain, and to my embarrassment in front of our class, highlighted my incorrect posture and poor spinal/cranial (head and back) alignment. It was a short assessment, but what I was taught, I never forgot, and am much more aware of my posture all these years later. I haven't had back pain again, (so far...watch this space...), and on a Nintendo Wii ™ machine, after the balance and posture assessment, my 'Wii' age came up as younger than my real age, unlike some of my relatives (I hope they don't read this). (If you're not familiar with this, it's only fun really, but a great machine and does help to make you think about general health, diet, exercise, coordination, balance and posture). I assure you that Nintendo™ aren't paying for the free ad, and I have no relatives in the firm. Seriously though, I mention it because like many of the complementary therapies, I don't have any good evidence, but based on experience, and from watching other people, some with neurological diagnoses, it can improve, for some, help with getting back muscular and coordination skills. Anyway, I put my success on the Wii™ machine down to my encounter with the Alexander technique teacher, despite it being brief and long ago.

The Parkinson's Disease Society acknowledge the lack of sound evidence but suggest that the Alexander technique may help people with PD to improve coordination, balance, fatigue and the tremor. They do warn that where practitioners are not regulated by law, for example in the UK, it is important to check the person has a valid qualification, and they recommend checking the following websites for information on this and generally on the technique: Alexander Technique International www.ati-net.com; Interactive Teaching Method Association www.alexandertechnique-itm.org; Society of Teachers of the Alexander

Technique (STAT) www.stat.org.uk.

While there isn't much evidence to associate claimed benefits of the Alexander Technique with specific neurological conditions, the anecdotal experiences of people concerning relief from stress, anxiety, sleep problems and widespread muscle pain and problems with gait and mobility mean that it does offer another potential option to consider for many. As with all interventions, discuss it with your consultant before commencing the therapy.

Aromatherapy

I should declare at the outset here that my wife, Sioux, is an aromatherapist, and a 'therapeutic masseuse' as well as having been a Practice Nurse, and now a Tissue Viability Nurse (specialist in wound care). She is trained for both complementary therapies with a recognised college belonging to a nationally well-reputed professional body, the importance of which has been emphasised (see under 'Acupuncture'). When she qualified in aromatherapy and therapeutic massage, she was working at a 40-bed specialist facility for young people with neurological conditions and these included all the conditions that have been the focus of this book. The facility was pleased to allow Sioux to offer this treatment to residents and the take up was high. Often people just asked for a foot or head massage, with or without special oils. But sometimes they went in for a neck and shoulders, back or whole body massage.

It's important that I do declare this personal interest, because when I talk about the effect this service had in the home, clearly I have a bias. There is, as I have emphasised with regard to complementary therapy generally, little evidence to support these anecdotal claims. But if anecdotes are the best evidence we have, that's what we may have to rely on though cautiously. Anyway, I worked at this place as well at the time, and I did feel despite my efforts to remain impartial that fairly quickly there was a change of atmosphere in the home in response to Sioux's healing hands. One of the problems, referred to earlier, associated with nursing in a care home is that there is often a lack of physical contact with patients. I mentioned in the previous section that we nurses no longer lift people, to protect our backs, but we do 'moving and handling' using hoists, slide sheets and other apparatus.

Added to that is the fear that touching people maybe misinterpreted - a justified fear perhaps - and that there might be allegations of sexual harassment. However well-intended these developments maybe, one down side is this potential starvation of physical contact, so important in ordinary life, and particularly when people feel unwell or isolated or fearful and anxious or frustrated. Our residents tended to experience all of those feelings frequently. Of course, inappropriate physical contact, especially unwanted, but also just not tactfully done, is arguably much worse than no contact at all and so many nurses and carers are appreciative of that. They opt just not to touch people at all... the safer bet.

Aromatherapy and therapeutic massage served to break down this barrier, providing gentle and firm, tender and professional, appropriate skin contact between the therapist and the patient, resident or client, depending on your favourite terminology for the people we strive to care for. Our visiting physician commented that he was prescribing less medication for sleep problems, to control aggression, and to alleviate anxiety and depression among the residents. You may think that his claim would be easy to check out, but really, it is difficult. There are all sorts of potential confounding factors to consider. Maybe he had already prescribed so much, everyone nearly, was on these medications, he didn't need to prescribe any more.

All right, apart from whether they were being prescribed less, maybe they weren't being given out as much. Is that to do with the aromatherapy, or was it because it was spring, then summer when this all happened, and people felt a bit better because of the sunlight or just not having to be cooped indoors so much? And if the pattern continued into autumn and winter, maybe courses staff had been on about managing these problems had helped them to come up with different strategies rather than resort to medication as they had done over six months previously. In that time maybe residents had deteriorated and were becoming more drowsy and less active and so less difficult to manage behaviourally without pharmaceutical input. It would be hard to rule out these possible explanations as challenges to the claim that the aromatherapy was responsible for less of this medication being prescribed or administered.

But most of us were convinced anyway that the aromatherapy had made a big positive impact. Quite apart from easing these psychological problems associated with neurological disease such as anxiety, depression, and aggravation and so on, there seemed to be reduced chorea in some of the people with Huntington's disease and easier movement in the limbs of people with Parkinson's disease. Sometimes the phenomena of 'freezing' discussed in the section on Parkinson's disease seemed to be overcome by a brief hand massage, which may have worked by just diverting attention momentarily.

Then the staff began to complain that they were just as stressed out as the people they were caring for, and asked for the service to be extended to them. On a trial basis the home allowed this, and soon the manager commented that there was a noticeable reduction in staff sickness and absence levels. This was attributed to the aromatherapy and felt to be worth keeping going. Staff members said that the treatment left them much more able to stay calm and patient when dealing with residents who were acting in normally socially unacceptable ways as a result of their conditions. Some suggested that the reason they were tending to give out less medication to residents for their aggressive episodes was that they were not perceiving it as such a problem to deal with. This led to interesting and slightly scary discussions about how much medication is given to residents to help staff rather than to help the resident directly. Answering this, and the question about whether we could be sure that reduced staff sick time was related to the aromatherapy and massage would have been just as difficult as the one on the reduction of prescriptions, with just as many potentially confounding factors.

So, what is aromatherapy then? Well, it utilises what are known as 'essential oils' that are derived from widely diverse plants and flowers. They can be inhaled (hence 'aroma') or applied in creams or dropped into bathwater to relax in. Most often though they are massaged into the skin by an expert aromatherapist. The oils are purported to contain active chemical properties that bring about mental and physical change. That is probably difficult to refute in many of them, because there is certainly some potential for harm if taken inappropriately. Many are dangerous to swallow, and they must be diluted before being applied to skin. Some people can have allergic reactions to the oils.

Once again, as with all complementary therapies, it is important to check with a doctor before venturing into treatment with aromatherapy and to ensure that the therapist is a member of a reputable professional organisation, particularly in countries where the practice is not regulated by law. Caution is particularly important in pregnancy and with conditions such as epilepsy or high blood pressure, asthma and diabetes. The doctor may advise you that some aromatherapy treatment is contraindicated (not to be taken in conjunction) with some medication that you are prescribed. But in some contraindicated conditions such as those mentioned above, it maybe possible for the therapist to carry out the massage with innocuous oil, and so, again, it is worth liaising with the doctor and the aromatherapist.

The following website is useful: www.aromatherapycouncil. co.uk.

Now, here's a point. You might think that with a wife seeming to make such a difference to so many people with those healing hands, I could be sure that at home, all those tensions of the day would be eased. Let me assure you that isn't the case. There is a saying, 'the cobblers kids are worst shod', or if that doesn't make sense to your colloquial dialect, how about 'the shoemaker's son always goes barefoot'.

Art Therapy

I have worked in many places that provide 'art therapy' allegedly, but the truth is, those of us who tried to run it had no formal training, and it was just a case of handing out big sheets of paper, paints and brushes, and other methods of application, then putting pinafore's around the resident to try and protect clothing, plastic sheeting around the floor, and saying, off you go, do your own thing. It tended to be messy and a lot of fun, and we saw all the range of human emotions expressed over time. And what could be wrong with that? It certainly seemed better to do it naively than just say, 'We don't do that because we're not trained and don't know much about it'.

According to the British Association of Art Therapists, art therapy is a 'form of psychotherapy that uses art media as its primary mode of communication'. Nicely put, what an art therapist does is try to facilitate the person to change and grow and personally develop as far as possible through their expression using art materials. It can be particularly helpful to people who just can't express themselves verbally or any other way for psychological reasons.

A range of art methods can be used. One approach uses an ancient art known as Batik. A piece of cloth or linen, let's say white, is dipped partially into a bath of dye, the lightest colour that is going to be used. Then when the cloth is dried it is white in a part, and another part is the colour of the first dye, let's say yellow. Now, hot wax is applied over an area that needs to remain white, and an area that needs to remain yellow. You see, you have to have a good idea of what end result you are aiming for, before you begin. After the wax dries hard, you dip the cloth in the next bath of dye, say light green, being just a bit darker than the yellow. Wax over the bit you want to keep green, and so on. Each time you dip the cloth in the new dye, the parts waxed over preserve the colours dyed onto the cloth the previous times.

The suitability of this method for people with a neurological disorder depends on the cognitive ability of the person, and their dexterity. You do need the ability to concentrate and persevere. And working with hot wax carries safety issues obviously. For the right people it can be relaxing, mesmerising and fun, and can be done singly or as a group. I hate to say, it tends to count out a lot of people with deteriorating disease. It's just too ambitious. I just mention it because for those individuals assessed as suitable, it can be so very absorbing and rewarding, and it helps to demonstrate diversity within the art therapy.

Using painting as a medium tends to be more accessible within our field, and this can be extremely expressive, fun and rewarding. It's popular as well because the practical pressures associated with organising the rest of the day, and freeing up staff time are less than with other methods. It's a quick job to get the materials out, and someone who only has a short attention span can leave it and return to it some other time without problems.

People can make models with clay and 'plasticine' or when times are hard, out of dough. They can be painted too. A trip to a well selected beach can allow individuals or groups to build with sand. Fabulous models can be made and it can be as expressive to knock them down as to build them up. Papier-mache is easy to make with paper and paste, and again can be used to make models or masks.

Whatever the medium, art therapists, usually trained to Masters level, need to be able to facilitate and guide the creative artistic aspects, ensuring safety, and equally able to draw the psychotherapeutic benefits from the activity engagement, for the person. It is a three-way interaction, between the artist, the therapist and the art media, whereas psychotherapy generally is a two-way procedure between the client and the therapist. Some deal with children, people with learning disabilities, and also with career adults trying to draw out better management skills, and there are many other practical applications.

I feel that there should be greater pressure on homes caring for people with neurological disorders to employ qualified art therapies. It is true that there is a lack of hard evidence for the benefits of a skilful approach over unskilled 'art therapy'. But based on my observations and anecdotal evidence, they are difficult to deny. It may be weak, but the best evidence we have. Sometimes it can be justifiable to act on low-level evidence to provide a therapy that has no ill effects, and people anecdotly find very helpful, for a condition without effective treatment. For many people with Alzheimer's disease and other forms of dementia, art therapy is often said to enable a release of pent up and destructive emotions. In one of the fairly rare studies carried out to try to shed light on the effect of art therapy on people with Alzheimer's disease, a group at Sussex University back in 1999 reported two main findings. First, they claimed that even after one session, people became more relaxed and sociable than people who didn't have the therapy. And secondly they found that the participant's depression scores as they were rated by the people working with them, went down over ten weeks when the study was carried out. The researchers acknowledge that this is not conclusive evidence, but it is an encouraging support for what anecdotally seems to be a useful and worthwhile intervention.

Conductive Education

I briefly mentioned this therapy in the section on Parkinson's disease. It comes from Hungary and is sometimes called the 'Petö system', being developed in Budapest by Professor Andras Petö during the 1940s. He regarded movement disorder as a learning problem that could be rectified by re-learning with the aid of a skilled therapist or 'conductor'. It is used with children with cerebral palsy, and I have to say, it is controversial. There are people who feel they have gained movement skills and the ability to carry out everyday activities of living through the method, and there are others who say they have found the procedures to be exhausting and futile. Some say the underpinning rationale is fundamentally flawed. This is because it involves going over and over an action, repetitively learning it and training the nervous system to restructure in order to make the action achievable and natural. 'I can adapt, and change my neurological organisation to be able to do what others do naturally' seems to be the fundamental attitude needed to be adopted.

Those who disagree with that starting point tend to make the point that it is better to say, 'We can adapt the environment to accommodate the way I am'. I must say, I had a bad experience observing this approach with an adult who had cerebral palsy, and a learning disability. He was unable to speak and protest. It was a long time ago, and thankfully, doctors are now much more prone to being concerned with gaining consent than some seemed to be then. But this poor fellow had a spastic arm. For hours at a time, he was trained to move down into a 'normal' straighter position, and this was aided by splints. After months and months of this painful and distressing procedure (that was disputed by the instigators, but the fellow's family and I saw it that way) it was discontinued and his arm was immediately as tightly flexed as it ever had been. I was thinking that I might not recount that tale as things must have moved on, and no one puts people through that now, but combing the web, there are certainly people giving similar and much more recent accounts.

There are also many very positive encounters reported and obviously many people experience a gentle repetitive learning approach and seemingly with tremendous results. With Parkinson's disease, the repeated activity tends to be simple and easy, such as rolling over sideways in a lying down position. It could involve going from a sitting position to standing or walking. The activities including a warm up are individually designed, unique to every client. The idea is that tasks learned and practised over and over will be goal orientated and will be a part of the practical every day movements that the person needs to be able to perform to get through ordinary days more easily. It is education rather than a therapy.

The National Institute of Conductive Education have a helpful website with www.conductive-education.org.uk. Again, as I do keep pointing out with all the complementary therapies, an organisation such as this is important if you are thinking about accessing Conductive Education. It maybe just right for you as it is for many, but where it is not regulated such as in the UK, you need to be sure the 'conductor' is legitimate. I think that was the problem in the sad case I conveyed to you above, because even though the person leading the treatment was medically qualified, he did not seem an expert in what is potentially a damaging procedure, compared to practitioners obtaining positive life-changing results. The National Institute of Conductive Education promote the potential benefits of this therapy for the right people with neurological conditions apart from the two I have mentioned, including Multiple Sclerosis, Stroke, Acquired Brain Injury, General Motor Disorders and Apraxia.

Herbal Medicine

Conventional pharmaceutical medicines are often derived (originally) from plants and so the idea that herbs may possess curative, healing or relieving properties that can be utilised to treat or manage a range of human ailments might appear to make the two health paradigms comparable. But they are quite different. The assumption underpinning the value placed on drugs in Western medicine is that to be considered effective they must stand up to the gold standard test of evidence—the randomised controlled trial, or RCT. In a randomised controlled trial, a large group of people are selected to be representative of the kind of people that would benefit if the drug does have the effect hoped for. The group is then split randomly so that some are allocated to be given the drug and others either given a sham drug (a placebo, as explained earlier in the section on acupuncture) or nothing or the standard existing treatment.

In what is called a double blind trial, those given the new drug and those given a placebo don't know what they are taking. Also, those administering the drug don't know whether they are giving the patient a placebo or an active drug. This is to ensure that any difference in the groups afterwards isn't influenced by a keen physician or nurse, who transfers the subconscious belief that it will work to the patient. The RCT must work to establish that the only reason for the desired change if it occurs more often in the treatment group than the placebo group must be the drug being tested. There are checks to make sure the comparative groups are matched on the basis of similar ages, health state and so on. If say, in the test of a drug intended to lower blood pressure, it does happen that the average blood pressure of the treatment group after taking the medicine is lower than the average of the placebo group, that could happen by chance. So a statistical test is run to ensure that the difference is significant, and is therefore very unlikely to have occurred as a matter of luck.

I mentioned under the heading 'Aromatherapy' that I would be challenging the idea that complementary approaches should be subjected to this kind of trial. My argument is that this ruling out of all the possible influencing factors except the drug is alien to the assumptions that underpin most other fields of health interventions including herbal medicines. The success of the 'modern' western approach in dominating health care and criticism of complementary therapies that they do not have the backing generally of evidence derived from rigorous RCTs has led to trials being carried out on them. But so far the trials on the complimentary medicine tend to be weak, and have not been rigorously controlled. Consequently, claims about good effects shown in results could be due to chance(luck). Perhaps the groups that were compared had some thing different about them, such as one group being older or less healthy than the other, that might have explained the results, rather than effects being caused by the complimentary medicine. Unfortunately, I feel, (and yes, this is a personal view only) these attempts to evaluate complementary treatments by the standards of Western modern medicine serve to undermine them rather than support them. It will never work, because it misses the point. Would it make sense to try to measure sound in feet and inches? If a loud noise didn't register anything on a ruler, does that make it not a real sound after all? No, sound is different to distance, it has to be measured in decibels.

As the underpinning assumptions of complementary medicines and of Western approaches are different, I don't think you can criticise herbal medicine or aromatherapy or acupuncture etc, on the basis that RCTs carried out on them are inconclusive. That's still all just my view by the way, not widely shared. I think that most professionals do think that we'll only know if herbal medicine or homeopathy work if they do stand up to RCTs. But I just can't agree. The assumption underpinning a therapy such as herbal medicine is that you can't separate out the herb, the environment, and the therapist from all his or her enthusiasm. It is a holistic approach and all those factors and the whole treatment experience are part of the healing. Rather than rule out the power of suggestion and the placebo effect, why not utilise them.

At the end of the day, what is the treatment for if not to make the client feel better? And if he or she does feel better, does it make sense to try to apportion how much of the effect was contributed by the therapist's nice manner, a bit of chance, the herb and the comfort of the room? Yes, in Western medicine culture it does make sense to separate it all out. In other cultures it doesn't really, if you did establish that the herb didn't work on its own, that doesn't mean it isn't effective as part of the whole procedure. Think about it. In a RCT, it shouldn't make any difference who administers the drug. In Herbal medicine, it really does matter. Experience and personal communication skills are a part of the healing. I can't see what's wrong with that. They are very different approaches and need to be assessed in different ways.

Please be aware that I am not suggesting for a minute that herbal and the other remedies don't need to be assessed for effectiveness and monitoring. I do and I would argue that they need to be monitored much more carefully than they are currently in many countries. It's just that the RCT approach, which I feel works very well and is suited to pharmaceutical medicine, is not the right test for some of these approaches. The outcomes we tend to look for in medical treatments are objective that is, we can observe and measure the effects. So, if the treatment is to lower blood pressure, we can measure whether it has reduced it or not. But complementary medicine outcomes tend to be subjective rather than objective. So it has more to do with the experience of being treated and how the person is feeling about any change they perceive. So, I'm sure we need to look for other measures to assess those effects.

A medical doctor though, should consider the interventions objectively, to advise on whether there maybe any property in the remedies that is contraindicated for reasons to do with the medication his patient has been prescribed or the patient's medical condition. And so it is important that there is communication between patient/client, doctor and the complementary therapist. If you feel I might have contradicted myself, that's because there is a difference between assessment of the suitability of a treatment for an individual patient in a clinical situation, and assessment of the effect of treatments on large groups in a research situation.

Maybe you don't agree, and feel strongly that the RCT is a safe bet- and all approaches, medical and complementary ought to measure up. I can understand that view too. Just thought it maybe worth putting forward another perspective. Anyway, here's a bit more about the Herbalists' approach. He or she will spend some time talking and listening to you and building up a holistic view of you- your lifestyle, current health state and past medical history, and will note any medications you are taking currently. You are then likely to have a mixture of herbs made up, suited to you individually. They will be given to be taken as a herbal tea, or as drops or capsules. You may well be given advice about your lifestyle, how to change your diet, and a specific exercise regime might be recommended to you.

Herbalists do treat people for specific neurological conditions such as dementia and Parkinson's disease, and whatever the diagnosis, they can particularly address symptoms such as memory loss and depression as well as skin disorders and impaired digestion. There is a herbal remedy called ayurveda, which is said to work similarly to Levodopa, and if so, may well be a suitable treatment for some people with Parkinson's disease. Speaking of which, here's a few cautionary points that are emphasised by the Parkinson's Disease Society, on their website (address given at the end of the book). They remind us of the importance of talking to your doctor before taking herbal medicines and point out rightly that some herbal medicines can have serious unwanted effects and can alter the way your medication works. In pregnancy be sure to check with the doctor, some herbal remedies will be contraindicated. They remind us too that you need to make sure you know that the herbs come from a reliable source, with UK medicines and healthcare products regulatory agency (MHRA) having frequently found herb supplies to be contaminated. They suggest that your GP would be able to advise on any recent alerts.

Just as is frequently emphasised here regarding all complementary therapies, especially in countries or states where there is no specific legal regulation, it is important to check that any herbalist you see is suitably qualified. On 14th June, 2008 in the UK, an article for the Telegraph by their health correspondent Laura Donnelly reported that some patients have suffered liver and kidney treatments after taking herbal remedies and that at least one person has died. A government Department of Health report recommends that herbalists (and other complementary medicine practitioners) should be registered and monitored and should have statutory minimum qualifications. That, I do agree with, and I believe in the countries where there is no regulation yet, it will come about soon -that certainly seems to be the case in my own country, the UK.

There are several relevant web addresses at the end of the book to help gain more information on Herbal Medicine.

Homeopathy

I really can't get my head around homeopathy, I have to say. But I can tell you that my father who had a real aversion to taking medical treatments found relief for his occasional mild ailments in homeopathic remedies as do many people I know. What's puzzling to us people rather rooted in what we think is conventional medicine- western pharmaceutical treatments, is that as we understand things, the more you take of a substance, the greater the effect generally, for good or for bad. That's why you never take more than the stated dose because it will work too effectively on your body, and therefore make more than the therapeutic change aimed for, and perhaps give way to a fatal change.

But in homeopathy, which is more than 200 years old, having been developed by a German physician named Samuel Hahnemann, the principle seems to work the opposite way. The more diluted the substance is, the more effective it seems to be. How can that be? I really don't know. But from the Homeopath's point of view, the extremely dilute substances selected to match the client's symptoms seem to activate the healing power within the person's own body, rectifying imbalances. The substances forming the basis of the remedies come from plants animals and minerals. When I say 'extremely dilute' I really mean it. A drop of the apparently active substance is put into a mixture of alcohol and water (often around 90% pure alcohol and 10% water). But this varies. After a few weeks during which from time to time the mixture is shaken, it is strained and it forms the 'mother tincture'. Then a drop of this diluted mixture is put into another alcohol/water mixture (for example, one drop put into 99 drops) and shaken. This process maybe repeated say 6 times depending on the level of dilution required. It can be seen that by the 6th dilution there must barely be a trace of the original substance in the resulting solution.

What miniscule trace there is though apparently stimulates the body to heal itself. 'Homeo' means similar or same; and 'pathy' refers to illness or disease as in 'pathology' or pathological'. So the term refers to giving a substance capable of bringing about a similar health problem to the one experienced, but in such small doses it can't do harm, but will activate the immune system to work against the disease. (Dis- ease just means the body is not at ease). Ipecac for example, can cause vomiting. A drop of ipecac diluted down as explained above repeating the process 30 times, seems to stop vomiting for many clients.

Like most complementary therapists, Homeopathists will obtain an overall picture of their client's way of living, health and illness history, any medications they maybe prescribed, the person's diet and the level of exercise they take. They may make some recommendations about changes to this lifestyle. Homeopathic remedies usually are in the form of a pill, and tend to be given to address symptoms rather than to treat a medical diagnosis. There are some claims that homeopathic treatment can help to slow the process of neurological disorders such as Alzheimer's disease or Multiple Sclerosis. But generally this is not suggested, and rather, problems such as stress, anxiety and depression that are associated with the disease are targeted.

Whether or not you can accept how homeopathy works, it certainly sounds safe, as the substances are so incredibly dilute, with barely a molecule of the original substance in the solution soaked into the pill. But no therapy is safe in the wrong hands, and you must have become aware by now, due to my repeated complementary message that treatments are individually arrived at through collaboration between client and therapist. So you should not just take something because a friend or a relative has taken it and it works for them. And of course, you need to ensure that the therapist belongs to a well-reputed regulatory (self regulatory in many countries) organisation, and is suitably qualified. Some useful web addresses are given at the end of the book.

Hydrotherapy

Instinctively, relaxing almost weightlessly suspended in water, strikes me as therapeutic, and I think this natural attraction towards hydrotherapy is what has given it its place as one of the more mainstream complementary therapies. It is an umbrella term for therapies involving water including relaxing in a Jacuzzi, mineral baths, a whirlpool bath, a cold plunge, massage underwater and many other approaches. The different pressures and temperatures of the water and the activities guided or carried out by the therapist apparently work together to ease pain as experienced in conditions such as Multiple Sclerosis and in cramp; spasticity or paralysis following a stroke; and stiffness, as seen in Parkinson's disease; calm chorea as seen in Huntington's disease and reduces anxiety and depression as often associated with dementia. These are just a few examples of the claims about how helpful it can be in caring for people with Neurological disorders. More broadly, it is widely reported to be helpful in relieving the symptoms of arthritis and other orthopaedic conditions, reducing blood pressure and the effects of burns.

I am not aware of statutory regulations anywhere in the world that specify minimum qualifications for practitioners of hydrotherapy and so once again it is important to ensure that anyone who treats you is suitably qualified. In hospitals and other care settings where I have either worked or visited and where hydrotherapy is provided, it is common for the practitioners to be registered nurses or physiotherapists who have undertaken specialised training. You do need someone who understands neurological conditions well as well as the general principles of water therapy.

Some specialised facilities I have visited find that hydrotherapy is popular among clients with Huntington's disease. You have to work a little harder to move in water and its viscosity appears to impede the choric involuntary limb and body movements, while allowing determined actions requiring effort. And generally, people with problems coordinating muscle contractions to maintain balance find that the exercise of working against a suitable level of turbulence tones up the body rendering the constant counteractions we have to make to stay upright. The pressure of the water surrounding the body means that expanding the chest to breathe takes greater effort. If this 'hydrostatic' pressure is too great, it could harm someone with neurological impairment leading to weakened inter-costal (between the ribs) muscles. But a good assessment can ensure that for the right person the extra effort builds up the strength and improves breathing.

The evidence for these benefits is poor as is the case with many of the other complementary therapies. Again, we are rather reliant on anecdotal evidence, from those who treat people and those who are treated. The thing that probably makes me enthuse a little is the feel good factor that many people derive from just going into the water anyway, whether or not the specific claimed positive therapeutic effects are lasting. You can imagine, I'm sure, how someone with advanced deteriorating disease, whether just impairing muscle control or impacting on mood, and causing confusion and disorientation, might feel, to have moments out of the buzzing world, floating, no longer having to deal with gravity. Fabulous, it has to be beneficial, provided the therapist is legitimate and safe as being in water without good co-ordination and cognition is not without risks by any means.

Hypnotherapy

My friend who first studied a degree in psychology and then trained to practice hypnotherapy has a wealth of anecdotal evidence from clients to testify to his ability to improve their golf, cope well with stressful management situations and make well-considered business decisions under pressure. In particular, he has helped many people overcome their fears, especially of flying. He found a good demand from this and has attracted many people through recommendation rather than advertising. Apart from the hypnotherapy itself, he is so keen that he can't help but give out positive messages about coping with everyday stresses and maximising your potential. About making money, he asked me, are you sure that's so important to you?

'Name someone rich, whom you admire', he said. 'David Beckham' I answered without thinking. 'How did he get rich?' he asked. 'Football', I answered. 'And what would he have done if football hadn't have made him rich?' 'Football anyway', I guessed. 'Who knows? But yes, probably. And wouldn't The Beatles, John Paul George and Ringo have all played music whether or not the records were hits?' 'I guess so' I said. Well then, the success that you admire is finding what is you, and doing it. That increases the chances of happiness and of earning more. It's easier to work hard if you're doing what is really you'. It's just good to be near someone like that, I find, and to people with a deteriorating health condition, he tends to help them to keep focussed on what they can do, and what they can still participate in, and what new opportunities might have arisen to, for instance, slow down and have time to enjoy TV or parts of a book or look at the birds in the garden, that just weren't possible when life was a bit more hectic, rather than stay pre-occupied with limitations and discomforts that the disease presents.

You have to have a genuine knack to get away with this, and you have to believe it, I feel, because it can sound pretty glib, and even offensive if 'positive' statements are delivered clumsily. It's true of all the complementary therapies as I keep emphasising, and certainly very true in the case of hypnotherapy that you need to be in the hands of a well-trained and regulated expert. The 'Hypnotherapy Association' is an example of a self regulating body that maintain a register in my own country, the United Kingdom, and there are many similar bodies around the world. Do seek advice from your doctor or nurse about an organisation to trust in your own region or country if you are thinking about going in for hypnotherapy, who can recommend a good therapist to you.

Again, I have shown how a complementary therapy, in this case hypnotherapy, tends to have to rely on anecdotal evidence to support claims about its potential benefits, and sadly I can give you anecdotal evidence in the other direction also. I was at a public open air town celebration day some years back, when a hypnotist got up on a stage and drew a big crowd. A hypnotist doesn't necessarily practice hypnotherapy of course and this is just a cautionary tale about the misuse of hypnotism in the more general sense. He got the crowd to join their hands and then suggested that they would not be able to separate themselves. A fair proportion found that indeed, they couldn't pull their own hands apart. From these people that he had identified as 'susceptible', he picked half a dozen to come up on stage and he got them doing silly antics, making a fool of themselves and causing the crowd to roar with laughter. When he began bringing them back to their normal conscious level, it became apparent that one young lady wasn't coming back. She collapsed, and was taken to hospital, and was quite ill for some time. This girl had a history of depression and anxiety and epilepsy. She was certainly not a good candidate for his show.

It was an example of the misuse of a skill that can be powerful for good or for harm. So, that's why I'm a bit repetitive regarding all the therapies about doing your best to avoid people who aren't properly qualified, trained and monitored. You can only do your best of course because the self regulating bodies in most countries aren't regulated by statutory independent bodies in the way that doctors, nurses, physiotherapists and so on are governed legally. So be careful.

There are many people who support the claims made within hypnotherapy that a good therapist can help to treat a wide range of health problems, and with regard to the conditions we have been discussing can treat anxiety, low mood, Multiple Sclerosis specifically, sexual problems and generally build up confidence and self esteem where the problems associated with a neurological diagnosis exist. People with epilepsy though, schizophrenia and clinical depression maybe contraindicated and are advised to consult their doctor before presenting for hypnotherapy. I would strongly recommend doing that anyway, whether or not you have any history of these complaints.

Meditation and Visualisation

Visualisation and imagery, often referred to as 'guided imagery' is another complementary therapy that involves a practitioner in helping the client to build a very detailed picture of a calm, peaceful setting—a place of your own, a refuge to go to at will, and to create the illusory experience of 'being there' away from the stresses of realities faced in daily living. It can be practised as a sole therapy, or in conjunction with relaxation strategies or meditation. These can enhance the effect of guided imagery making it easier to 'access' and remain at the personal, private, mental location, for as long as is required.

In a demonstration session some years ago, I created a rather pleasant sunny and convincing setting for myself, and although I haven't been back, I do still benefit from that short isolated experience. The scene is a beach of very white powdery sand wafting in the gentle breeze. I am walking barefoot in shorts and T shirt and I can feel the heat of the sand on my feet. To the right of me are grassy dunes, and way ahead are leaning, stretching palm trees, while to my left, about 100 yards away, the blue and sparkling sea is lapping onto the beach. I can feel a trickle of perspiration running from my forehead, and I wipe it with the back of my left hand, and then lift the glass of iced lemonade to my mouth with my right hand. The taste is so refreshing. The sun is just a little too bright and its heat on my face makes me look for relief. As I pass the next dune on my right, a marble cave comes into view, and as I step into its entrance, I immediately feel the benefit of its cool shade. Standing there, I sip the lemonade and watch the sea slip forwards and backwards rhythmically along the shore. The sound is mesmerising and almost hypnotic, gradually absorbing all of my attention.

Well, I've kept that little 'place' ever since. It was a fabulous session, and I find I can quickly pay it a visit when sitting on a dentist's chair and in all sorts of situations where I'm not too comfortable or perhaps somewhat stressed. I find that I really feel those sensations, hear those sounds, 'see' the imagery (although, I don't know if I'm unusual, but I don't shut my eyes and I can equally well see the real physical world around me) and I can hear the sounds. I find this lasting legacy of a short informal demonstration eases toothache, headache and helps me with the short blast of stage-fright that I tend to get out of just before public speaking.

I am an amateur though and am only dabbling. If you are going to learn it properly, see your GP or specialist neurological nurse and get advice. Of course, this, like many of the complementary therapies can be as useful to carers as to the person with the diagnosis. They may give you guidance to help you develop techniques for yourself, or they may suggest someone who is a member of a reputable body. Don't go to a 'therapist' on the basis of an advertisement without a recommendation. That would be my advice. The person could well be dabbling like myself, and although they might not harm you, it would be what we in my corner of the world call a 'rip-off' (money wasted). But imagery can be negative and cause harm. Good thoughts can have a good effect on your physical body. It's mind over matter. Similarly, bad, or negative thoughts can have a detrimental physical effect.

Thinking of nice places whether real or made up as the one I described, and pleasant walks works for a lot of people. There are other ways to use imagery. People claim to have made physiological changes to the body by picturing organs, cells, the immune system imagined in all sorts of ways, in action, fighting disease, clearing blockages and so on. People picture their medication going around the body beating off tumours, or boosting the growth of neurones, and some report dramatic effects. There are anecdotal tales of women unable to produce breast milk, solving the problem by imagining an abundant flow. Less dramatically, I have been in situations where I feel I am about to burst if I don't find a urinal. By picturing the sphincter closing off the bladder, and the bladder itself becoming more relaxed and elastic, I have found that the sensation of urgency vanishes. Trouble is, not for long, but I'm sure with effort this could be perfected. I only think of it when desperate. (By the way, you can improve continence by exercising the 'pelvic floor' muscles, but you do need the guidance of the continence nurse for this. Incorrect attempts can make the problem worse).

Those who promote this therapy make numerous claims about its effectiveness in helping people including those with neurological disorders to reduce stress associated with the condition, calm fear and panic and anxiety. It is said to help with managing anger and pain, depression and problems with getting a good night's sleep. If you have these problems and find that this approach is effective for you, it could help you to reduce the amount of medications you take for the symptoms, and that in itself can be very positive, given that most medications are associated with at least some unwanted effects even if mild. With a bad toothache for example, I do, as I mentioned above find imagery reduces pain. But I tend to need some medication eventually. But I do end up taking much less than I would without this adjunctive therapy.

Music Therapy

As far as I know, I've never met anyone who didn't have some appreciation for some kind of music, and couldn't react to it in some way. I've met one or two people who struggle to follow the rhythm... and when they dance, the feet step randomly at intervals that seem to have nothing to do with what the percussionist or bassist is doing. A relative who was keen to dance the first waltz at his wedding spent a long time listening to various members of our family explain. 'Listen, one two three, one two three...'. He could hear the thump sound in the music, but after hearing one, seemed unable to predict the arrival of the next. He then attended lessons with a famous dance teacher, who had no more success than the family members at establishing when the feet should contact the ground. But, this is a person who loves music, and is an ardent fan of a well known band. He sings along, and sounds well in tune. If the drummer went out of time, he'd notice something was wrong.

I have other friends who step in time, without any problem, yet when they sing along, they're way out of tune. They're well aware of that, but they love it. Another friend is a professional musician. He taught someone who is deaf to play the guitar by feeling the changes in vibration through the sound box, and responding to them. He has become quite accomplished and obtains enormous pleasure from it. So I feel pretty confident that this appreciation of music is innate, inborn and universal. Taste in types of music of course is hugely varied. What stirs up happy or romantic or patriotic emotions in one individual maybe an annoying noise to another. Or maybe, it stirs up other passions such as anger or sadness. The music that we grow up to associate with our fun, carefree times, first romances, first car and first broken heart tends to hold that association with the feelings that go with those experiences through most of our lives, even if we forget the event that had caused the emotion initially.

For pretty much everyone then, music can be therapeutic and can help us to relax and unwind, or liven up and get into the party mood, become thoughtful, or help to evoke memories. There are some people I've known briefly in the past, and some places that I'm sure would be lost to me - I would never picture or think of again, except that when a certain record plays, I am transported back, and I'm sure you have similar experiences. Speaking of how music can help to retrieve memories, I remember when I was studying for my nursing final examination, I tried a personal experiment. Every time I read about the heart or blood or circulation, I played Elton John in the background. (Well, it was a long time ago!). When I studied bones and muscles, joints, tendons and ligaments, I had the Beatles. And to learn about the nervous system including the brain, I played Freddie Mercury with Queen. When the learning got too technical or if I came across facts that were new to me, I had to turn the music off and concentrate in silence, but for going over old stuff that I needed to drum into my head, or learn materials that didn't seem too hard and looking at diagrams and pictures, I found the music great.

When it came to the big stressful examination day, I took a look at each question and began writing the answers. Each time I struggled to recall aspects of anatomy and physiology, or what the appropriate care was in certain circumstances, I sat back, and began conjuring up the songs related to the relevant body system. It worked a treat! I had a question about a patient who had a duodenal ulcer. I got terribly stuck and couldn't think of the causes or treatments or advice to give for the future. It all came flooding back as I calmly stopped trying so hard to think of the answer, and 'listened' to Bruce Springsteen in my head.

In music therapy, music becomes the medium through which the client and the therapist communicate. In the course of a session, both tend to play a range of instruments, sing and listen to music. It's not a teaching session in which the client is trying to learn how to play or sing, but by freely performing, a range of percussive instruments, the expression of pent up thoughts and feelings can be released and communicated in a way that the normal channels such as talking or writing may not be able to facilitate.

Apart from improving helping to address psychological aspects such as self esteem, reducing stress, aiding memory and helping with problems to do with communication, it can be very helpful with increasing a range of movement, say, in limb movement impaired following stroke, and in movement disorders that we have discussed. Exercise can be much easier and less boring if done with music, enabling people with limited staying power to persevere a little more. Of course, the usual advice applies. Discuss your wish to take up music therapy with your doctor and seek a qualified therapist. This is important because a person with Parkinson's disease for example, maybe able to improve their gait, and ability to move the limbs freely with the aid of music, but not if it is not set at a carefully selected tempo for appropriate lengths of time with suitable intervals. Unless the therapist is skilled, the condition could be exacerbated rather than improved.

Pilates

Born in 1879, Joseph Pilates to whom the name of this complementary therapy is owed, is quoted as saying in 1956 at the age of 86—'I must be right. Never an aspirin. Never injured a day in my life. The whole country, the whole world, should be doing my exercises. They'd be happier'. Another of his claims is— 'In 10 sessions, you will feel the difference. In 20, you will see the difference. And in 30, you'll be on your way to having a whole new body'. These were taken from: www.pilatesforhealthyjoints.com where there are many more classic one-liners of his that are all remembered widely across the public domain.

It is a low-impact exercise formula that is claimed to be able to increase physical and mental health. It is fairly popular among some sports amateurs and professionals and dancers wishing to tone up mind and body, while anxious to avoid over-exertion and injury. It focuses on what are regarded as the 'core' muscle groups in the back and abdomen. Posture is said to improve as is agility and flexibility. Pilates applies eight principles. They are relaxation, routine, alignment, breathing, control, centring, precision and flowing movement. It's not an 'aerobic' form of exercise in the way that jogging and swimming are, but it does demand an exertion or effort.

Generally, Pilates is claimed to be able to help to reduce the stresses of daily living, relieve pain and tension and can help people go off to sleep. The improvements in posture and balance said to result from Pilates are apparently associated with a reduction in falls. It is reported that people with movement disorders such as Parkinson's disease can benefit by improving the communication between brain and the body, and the breathing exercise increases oxygen supply boosting energy.

Once again, it is a therapy that requires qualified teaching and guidance, and supervision to ensure that people, particularly those with neurological conditions such as Parkinson's, find a level to work at that is therapeutic and avoid over-exertion. The Pilates Foundation and the Pilates Institute are examples of organisations that may recommend accredited and suitably trained teachers. It is important to let them know of course that you have a neurological diagnosis, and to seek advice about considering taking up Pilates from your GP (family doctor), before going along.

Reflexology

The ancient practice of reflexology is based on a notion that the whole body is represented on the soles of the feet, and to some extent on the hands, with specific foot 'zones' relating to particular body organs and areas. I had decided many years ago that this was a therapy I would have to decline, because my feet are so ticklish that I cannot allow anyone to get near them. My children grew up knowing that they should never try it, even for a joke. They are SO sensitive, (my feet, not my children) I really can't help it, I just kick out immediately if anything gently brushes against the underside of either foot. I warned a podiatrist about this when I went to have my ingrown toe nails removed. He told me that injections each side of the nails would be painful, but I wasn't bothered by them, but did keep reminding him not to touch the underneath of the feet. Then he did it, and quick as a flash, his chin caught the reflex reaction.

So when a reflexologist told me she could manipulate my soles, I begged to differ. I told her how fast and automatic my ticklish reactions are, and that people tend to get bruised if they get anywhere near either of my feet, and she saw this as a challenge. It seemed unbelievable to me that within minutes she was working the soles of my feet like dough, without stimulating any untoward reaction. In fact, the experience was incredibly calming and relaxing. It seemed a shame to let her stop. Fantastic, I have to report.

And as we have generally seen with the complementary therapies, the evidence supporting the effects is largely anecdotal and subjective, like my account. A lot of people of course, value this kind of evidence more than the results of experimental trials, believing that 'the proof of the pudding is in the eating'.

There are ten energy zones running through the body according to the principles underpinning reflexology and the therapist works on the feet and sometimes the hands to unblock channels that have become hampered by disease or imbalance. When these channels are unblocked the energy flows more freely again and health is restored to some extent. Therapists claim to be able to clear unwanted effects of toxins in the body that may build up because of medicines used to treat neurological conditions, and to help with problems such as constipation that maybe associated with the diagnoses, stimulate the firing of natural chemicals in the brain.

Reflexologists suggest that by working a thumb in a skilled way over the area of the foot that relates to the diaphragm and solar plexus in the body, tremor in Parkinson's disease can be alleviated. This seems to be (I'm a complete layman with regard to this) a curve stretching from the inner to the outer edges of each foot at a level just below the ball of the foot. The area corresponding with the brain by the way is at the top of each big toe, and the inner aspect of each foot has a relationship with the spine. Clearly there's a lot more to it than that and you need an expert to tell you. There is a great deal of anecdotal evidence about people with conditions such as Amyotrophic Lateral Sclerosis finding that over time, benefits of treatment are experienced.

Depending on which country you live in, you may or may not be able to access reflexology through the health service, but either way, you do need to check with your doctor that it is suitable for you, and that if you do attend, the reflexologist is suitably trained and monitored. There is a web address that maybe useful at the end of the book.

Reiki

Reiki is all about physical (the body) mental (the mind) and spiritual (the soul) healing and restoring balance or equilibrium. This is seemingly achieved by channelling universal energy known as 'chi' to balance the seven major 'chakras' in the human body. Reiki seems to strengthen the bond between body and mind, capitalising on the mind's power to influence physical self-healing. It is regarded as particularly safe by promoters of the therapy because of its non-invasive nature. Like many of the complementary therapies it is often promoted as an adjunct to medical or other treatment. The therapy is said to bring about a sense of inner peace and calm in people with a wide range of illnesses or long term impaired health conditions including neurological disorders. Stress can be relieved and emotions brought under control. Damaged tissue in the body can be nourished and healed apparently and a 'life force energy' feeds and revives the soul.

More specific claims include the ability of Reiki to channel energy to parts of the brain that produce or regulate dopamine and to affect the blood-brain barrier so that the effect of medication intended to treat the brain is enhanced. Depression that may accompany any of the conditions that we have discussed can be alleviated through the sense of well-being that is reported in association with Reiki. I had a colleague who took up the practice of Reiki and certainly reports from people he treated were very positive. After I moved away from the area, I was speaking to him on the phone once and he offered me some therapy over the phone. I had no idea this was believed to be possible but my colleague couldn't understand my amazement. 'I can focus the energy, and it's your mind that will take control and cause your body to heal itself. Why shouldn't that be possible over the phone?' I turned him down, but perhaps I shouldn't have. Anyway, it does seem that Reiki at a distance is fairly widely practiced.

If you do decide to consider Reiki you should check that the therapist is qualified and recognised by a reputed governing body, depending on the country you live in. In my own country for example, I might seek a recommendation from a GP or a friend and then check that the practitioner is registered with an organisation promoting good practice and integrity such as the PRHT (the Practitioner Register for Holistic Therapies), a member organisation of the BCMA, the British Complementary Medicine Association.

Shiatsu

Shiatsu has similar aims as Reiki, above, in that it seeks to cultivate the body's own self-healing power by bringing about harmony in the flow of energy or 'Chi' or 'Ki', resulting in a healthier mind, body and spirit. This harmony is achieved by a different means though, and involves applying pressure with thumbs, hands, elbows, knees and feet. Treatment is given on a soft mat on the floor usually and also involves stretching and rotating arms and legs and joints. The treatment, again, like Reiki, despite the great difference in its form, is said to support and nourish 'life-force', and relieve tension, increase self-awareness and generate overall well-being. Shiatsu can apparently be used as a preventative therapy for many conditions, including stroke, in the context of this book. It is also claimed to treat health crises, with regard to wide ranging health conditions.

It is important to choose a therapist who is properly qualified and a member of a reputable body that maintains and monitors standards, as incorrect practice of this therapy could result in injury and worsening of a neurological condition. The web addresses of the Shiatsu Society, and of the European Shiatsu Foundation, to which the Shiatsu Society is affiliated are provided at the end of the book. The Shiatsu society states that all its practitioners are full members. and have a minimum of 3 years training. After graduation they are all assessed. It claims to maintain a strict code of ethics by which the practitioners must abide and that membership provides them with full insurance.

These organisations maybe useful but your physician or specialist neurological nurse maybe able to help you identify an appropriate practitioner locally, in your own country.

Shiatsu is claimed to help to relieve emotional problems such as stress, anxiety and depression. Muscular tension, neck and back ache, arthritis and posture problems as well as injuries to joints such as sprains are also said to be eased by Shiatsu. People report finding relief from diarrhoea and constipation, acid reflux or 'heartburn', nausea and impaired appetite, and also colds, flu, asthma and other breathing related conditions. Shiatsu is said to help with headache and migraine, sleep problems and a lack of energy. Any of these benefits maybe of help to people with a degenerative neurological illness and specifically, Shiatsu is regarded by many as a therapy that can help to stabilise a condition such as Multiple Sclerosis, and help to improve circulation to paralysed areas following a stroke. Practitioners advise clients to seek their input as early as possible following a stroke and also claim that they can help to reduce the chances of having a stroke for those who are at risk. Anecdotal evidence abounds with some people claiming fairly dramatic improvements in memory and partially restored personality in Alzheimer's disease.

It is not easy to assess how lasting these reported effects tend to be and while I think it is important not to have too high an expectation of any treatment for a degenerative neurological diagnosis, the belief that you can be helped seems to play a major part in the relief of symptoms, and also the general sense of well-being reported so widely in association with Shiatsu and other hands-on, invigorating complementary therapies must make the symptoms easier to deal with.

Tai Chi

There are many forms of Tai Chi but 'Tai Chi Chuan' is the Chinese martial art form that is practised widely for health, and so when many people consider the form that may help them to maximise physical mental and spiritual health and refer to 'Tai Chi', they do mean 'Tai Chi Chuan'. It can be practised at a variety of levels ranging from simple movements and meditation to a serious martial art. For laymen like myself when it comes to Tai Chi, the easily recognisable form is known as the hand form. I will never forget the first time I witnessed this. I woke up in Hong Kong at around 6 am one morning and decided to leave my hotel and have a good walk before breakfast, prior to attending a conference on how to measure 'quality of life'.

You might well wonder why anyone would want to try to measure a seemingly vague concept such as 'quality of life'. But it is very relevant to professionals who are seeking to establish which interventions should be available and recommended to people with all sorts of conditions and in my case, people with neurological disorders. If for example, a treatment is shown to reduce chorea in Huntington's disease, or tremor in Parkinson's disease, or improve memory in Alzheimer's disease for example, from the observations and measurements made by a neurologist or other health professional, does that necessarily mean that the treatment has made life better as the person experiences it? In my experience of talking to people who have had treatments the answer is often 'no, not necessarily'.

And if a treatment does add to the quality of a person's life, despite failing to reduce tremor or chorea or improve memory, how could you convince a National Health Service of the benefits, so that there is an incentive to fund the intervention? Does sitting in a Jacuzzi improve the quality of life more than sitting in a 'snoozalem' room which is a special relaxation room with gentle sensory stimulation involving soft lights? With limited funds which would be the better investment to equip a specialist neurological facility with? You have to have some measure of 'quality of life' to be able to try and answer those questions.

Well, that was my excuse for being in Hong Kong, and as I reached the park opposite my hotel before 6.30 am, I was amazed to see crowds of people of all ages, dressed up ready for school or work, or apparently retired, and mums with young babies, all making slow, controlled and artistic hand, limb and body movements in silence. Most had stopped to do this, some individually, and some in small or large groups. Some of the groups had an obvious leader or instructor at the front checking that everyone was copying the motions correctly. But other people did not stop, and instead carried on walking holding their satchels or briefcases making the postural and hand gestures as they progressed along towards their destination. I got back to the hotel after a circular trip by around 8 am, and still in streets as well as parks there were many people carrying out Tai Chi.

Even watching the activity gave me a deep sense of calm and spiritual well-being. It truly is a beautiful sight. Since then, I have seen increasing numbers of people taking this up in Western parks, but as yet these represent a minority, whereas in Hong Kong and many areas of China it is a very mainstream pursuit.

There are claims that Tai Chi can dramatically reduce the numbers of falls among people with Parkinson's disease. Also that people with Multiple Sclerosis and other neurological conditions affecting movement and balance can vastly improve posture and breathing and general vigour, and reduce depression through the practice of Tai Chi. Whether or not the claims can be justified through substantial evidence, it is hard to argue after watching these people, from children to octogenarians and beyond, that they aren't benefitting in some way through increased flexibility, and suppleness. If it is so relaxing to watch, surely doing it will help to reduce the pressures and stresses that face us whether or not we have or are caring for someone with a neurological disorder.

To help you with finding out more about Tai Chi if you wish to, a potentially useful website is provided at the end of the book – it is a British website but has international links.

Yoga

This is another 'holistic' (whole body, mind and soul, all encompassing) approach to well-being. I think I'm fairly fortunate in that as I naturally have a slightly meditative disposition. And I put it down to that I have learned generally to put troubles down until in a position to do something about them. At home, I don't tend to ruminate over matters that need to be sorted out at work, and at work I'm not consumed with problems that have a solution at home. Money problems I tend to deal with at the bank. But as a nurse-lecturer, I try to play a supportive role and I often find that students who have most difficulties with the course have a real problem with deciding when and where to deal with issues in a practical way.

Something upsetting may have happened at home and it becomes an issue during work time or when trying to write an essay. I don't mean there's something wrong if a real disaster happens and it impacts on all areas of life; that would just prove you're human. But then you have to decide whether you're fit to be at work or not. Similarly, they might fail an essay that has to be re-written, and they tell me that they're losing sleep at night. That won't get the essay written.

I have found that being pre-disposed to a meditative mentality does help to unwind and stay focussed on what the next thing is that needs to be done, rather than spending energy mulling over and over on what might happen, how cross I am with someone, how let down I feel, or how humiliated I am by some kind of sense of failure. I don't find that any of those thoughts tend to solve the troubles.

I don't formally practice Yoga but I have been to some beginner's sessions provided by a member of a fairly local Buddhist community. It is not only associated with Buddhism but also Hinduism and Jainism. We didn't get to try any of the postures that people often think of in connection with Yoga, but instead were guided to sit on a low stool and become increasingly aware of our breathing. I visualised the air around me moving into my mouth (you should breathe in with your nose and out via your mouth, but I can't do it. I'm a complete mouth breather... three attempts to breathe in via my nose and I'm gasping for air) and down into my lungs, and back out, rhythmically and smoothly. I found soon that I was thinking of nothing else, and nothing else mattered. Every now and then a thought crept in. I pictured the thought being encapsulated in a bubble and then drifting away.

I have found that without any formal attempt to meditate, I can sometimes do this with pain. I can feel it, but the feeling is in a bubble, drifting off separately from me. I emphasise... sometimes I can do it, and it is for a limited period. Eventually, if a toothache is bad my capacity to send it drifting off in a bubble is exceeded. Practice would fix that.

In more advanced Yoga classes people are taught to practice call and response chanting, proper meditation (that is, beyond my dabbling level) or listening to the instructor reading inspirational material. Some people use Yoga mainly to gain physical benefits, and while they might warm up beforehand with exercises to prepare muscles, joints and tendons, they might not necessarily meditate. And some do Yoga purely for spiritual growth, or to stay mentally in shape, while others do it to feel great. It's very personal.

The general benefits implied so far could certainly be regarded as relevant to most people with a neurological diagnosis and their carers. But more specifically, in Multiple Sclerosis, Yoga is claimed to help in three main areas—fatigue and heat intolerance; impaired coordination, muscle spasms and sensory loss or numbness in the limbs and problems to do with balance and flexibility. In Parkinson's, there is a wealth of anecdotal evidence testifying to improvement in symptoms and in the ability to come to terms with having the condition. Mobility, flexibility, emotional well-being and general level of quality of life are all reported to improve with Yoga. Yoga is said to reduce artherosclerosis (the development of plaques within the walls of arterial blood vessels) and therefore cut down on the risk of heart attacks and strokes, and in those who have suffered a previous stroke, cut the risk of a further incident. Similarly, there are accounts from people with Motor Neuron Disease testifying an improvement in balance, movement and in breathing and swallowing using Yoga as an adjunct to speech and language therapy.

The Yoga beginner's sessions I mentioned attending, were attended by people with Huntington's disease and their carers. They certainly seemed to reach a general positive consensus regarding the benefits on anxiety, stress, involuntary movement and on being able to escape from as one person with HD told me, 'being trapped in this body'.

So there are many complementary therapies, and only relatively few are briefly outlined above. And within each or closely related to each there are usually numerous fields. For example, I outlined acupuncture, but not acupressure which is similar but uses pressure as the name suggests rather than fine needles.

Throughout the discussion, the importance of seeking advice from your doctor or specialist nurse on whether seeking a particular therapy maybe a good idea, is emphasised, as is seeking out a qualified practitioner. Some therapies that involve massage or other invasive interventions demand particular caution because delicate, weakened muscles in a condition such as Motor Neuron Disease could easily be harmed by non-expert handling.

Other than that, it is a matter of personal preference, perhaps initially based on recommendation and then on personal experience, whether a particular therapy is right for you or not. If you find an intervention that either relieves symptoms or helps you to deal with them or both, and leaves you feeling much better than before, I'd say it's an indication that it's good for you. This is true for both the person with the diagnosis and the carer. Ideally, you will feel after a treatment, that you've stepped out of all the trouble and discomfort the diagnosis brings with it for a while, and will feel you've been pampered, and spoiled, and ready to take life on with a bit more enthusiasm.

If you do find a treatment that does all that for you, I'm not too sure I'd be over concerned about any evidence in its favour being largely anecdotal, rather than having the support of randomised controlled trials (experimental evidence). The proof of the pudding I'd say, is in eating.

Conclusion

Thank you so much for getting this far with this book. We do have a remarkable central nervous system with so many incredible functions making us able to sense and react to the world around us; communicate with others; think, imagine and dream, and do many incredibly complex tasks so easily that we take a lot of it for granted. It is the system that is deeply entangled in our very being, giving us our sense of who we are. Anything we do that conveys our love to those dearest to us depends on our central nervous system.

And so when this system is impaired the impact on us and those nearest and dearest can be devastating. The task of caring for someone giving off inappropriate body language, acting out of character and who often may seem ungrateful is an enormous challenge although many do find it most rewarding. It can help if formal carers including qualified nurses and Health Care Assistants, therapists of all kinds, physicians and social workers, can find ways to think and talk to informal carers such as spouses, and other family members, neighbours and friends about what the problems are and how they might best be approached, in a shared language.

That's what this book has sought to contribute towards. Not to address all the issues or give answers to specific problems.

You do need to work together as a team. Everyone in the team has some relevant expertise. Above all, the family caregiver and the person who has the diagnosis have the expertise concerning the real problems being faced. Solutions have to be individualised to stand a chance of working. There is further expertise to draw on also voluntary organisations and other support that maybe helpful. I enclose a list of some of those at the end of the book.

Finally, I really do understand if your criticism of this book is that I have taken what seems to be a rather pessimistic view of neurological conditions and the effect they can have on individuals and their families and friends. That is probably because I've been keen to address aspects that are particularly difficult. And I find that a lot of people going through a very hard time, maybe reaching a point where it seems impossible to stay on top emotionally. If they feel that the heaviness of the load they're bearing is acknowledged and appreciated, their energies are revived. And so, I haven't held back from making reference to the severity of the impact people can experience. There are many positive things that can be said about living with a neurological diagnosis whether from a carer or care-receiver's perspective.

But I think that if I'd have given this the emphasis, it could be offensive. You can tell me that you don't let the disease define you; or you find life has more meaning and so on. That's great and I know many share those feelings about the changes that the condition brings about. But it does have to come from you really. I can't tell you, 'Keep your chin up; think positive; it's enriching'. That would be an awful emphasis coming from me, as a health professional. It is often seen that people - couples for example, do find that they feel closer sometimes; people have more time to do the simple, enjoyable and meaningful things in life. And I have referred to this, but not dwelt on it.

Whether you are caring informally as a partner, family member, neighbour or a friend, and whether directly and intimately, or at a distance, keeping an eye on the care or whether you are caring as a health professional, you must look after yourself, and be honest in your assessment of how well you can continue to manage what you are doing. Keep in touch with various members of health and social care professions and debrief. Leave them in no doubt about what you can manage and what is stretching you. Make sure your days and weeks have breaks, entertainment and socialising included in them.

Caring can be very rewarding it's true, and can be fun and fulfilling. It can also be pretty draining. I've been writing from a nursing experience, but I do have personal experience as well. I say that in the hope that the next sentence won't sound too aloof. Life may have changed, with all your life plans. It's different to how you might have envisaged it, but it's not over. And you do make a difference; your input counts. If you're not convinced that what you spend your time doing with or for the person you care for, at whatever level, directly or indirectly, makes a difference, have another look at the section near the beginning of this book, under the heading 'plasticity'. Then congratulate yourself for doing your best. That's all we can do, we're just human beings after all.

My very best wishes.

References

1. Alzheimer's Society (2009), What is Alzheimer's? www.alzhe imers.org.uk

2. Baddeley, A, Hitch, G. (1974). Working Memory, In G.A. Bower (Ed.), The psychology of learning and motivation: advances in research and theory Vol. 8, pp. 47-89), Academic Press, New York.

3. Barone P, Zappia M, Quattrone A. (2006). MRI Imaging of Middle Cerebellar Peduncle Width: Differentiation of Multiple System Atrophy from Parkinson's Disease, Radiology, 239(3): 825-830.

4. Department of Health (UK); (2009), Living well it dementia: a National Dementia Strategy, HMSO, London.

5. Department of Health (UK); (2007) National Stroke Strategy, HMSO, London.

6. Debouverie M, Pittion-Vouyovitch S, Louis S, Guillemin F. (2008). 'Natural history of multiple sclerosis in a population-based cohort'. European Journal of Neurology, 15(9):916-921.

7. Factor S, Weiner, W. (2002), Parkinson's Disease: Diagnosis and Clinical management, Desmos; New York.

8. Greenfield, S. (2008). ID: The Quest for Meaning in the 21st Century, Sceptre.

9. Greenfield, S. (2000). The Private Life of the Brain. Allen Lane.

10. Greenfield, S. (1998). The Human Brain: A Guided Tour, Basic Books.

11. Hardin S, Schooley, B. (2002). A Story of Pick's Disease: A Rare Form of Dementia, Journal of Neuroscience Nursing, 34(3):117-22.

12. Highfield, R. (2009). In your face, New Scientist, 201(2695): 29-32.

13. Hofstadter, D. (2007). I am a strange loop, Basic Books, New York.

14. Kertesz, A. (2006). Progress in Clinical Neurosciences: Frontotemporal Dementia – Pick's Disease, Canadian Journal of Neurological Sciences 32(2)141-148.

15. Lee M, Shin B, Kong J, Ernst E. (2008). Effectiveness of Acupuncture for Parkinson's disease, Movement Disorders, 15; 23 (11): p1505-1515.

16. McGuire E, Gadian D, Johnsrude I, Good C, Ashburner J, Frackowiak R, Frith C. (1999). Navigation-Related Structural Change in the Hippocampi of Taxi Drivers, Proceedings of the National Academy of the United States of America; 97 (8):4398-4403.

17. Mental Capacity Act (2005) Department of Health, HMSO, London.

18. Miller, G. A. (1956). The magical number seven, plus or minus two: Some limits on our capacity for processing information. Psychological Review, 63, 81-97

19. Motor Neuron Disease Association. (2009). Different types of MND, www.mndassociation.org , visited 02 03 2009.

20. Multiple Sclerosis Society. (2009). About MS, www.mssociety. org.uk visited 02 03 2009.

21. National Institute on Aging. (2009). Alzheimer's Disease factsheet, US Department of Health and Human Sciences, San Francisco.

22. National Institute of Neurological Disorders and Stroke-www.ninds.nih.gov

23. Nicoletti G, Fera F, Condino F, Auteri W, Gallo O, Pugliese P, Arabia G, Morgante L,

24. Pablo M, Carmen R, Belen F. (2008). Specific patient-reported outcomes for Parkinson's disease:analysis and applications, Expert Review of Pharmacoeconomics and Outcomes Research, 8(4): 401-418.

25. Parkinson's Disease Society. (2008). Drug treatment of Parkinson's disease, for people living with Parkinson's, PDS, London; (Downloadable at http://www.parkinsons.org.uk/ PDF/B013_September_web.pdf).

26. Pick's Disease Support Group, www.pdsg.org.uk

27. Pierre N. Tariot, MD; Martin R. Farlow, MD; George T.

Grossberg, MD; Stephen M. Graham, PhD; Scott McDonald, PhD; Ivan Gergel, MD; for the Memantine Study Group (2004). Memantine Treatment in Patients With Moderate to Severe Alzheimer Disease Already Receiving Donepezil, Journal of the American Medical Association. 291:317-324.

28. Pollard, J. (2008). Hurry up and wait, Boston.

29. Romero E, Cha G, Verstreken P, Ly C, Hughes R, Bellen H, Botas J. (2008). Suppression of neurodegeneration and increased neurotransmission caused by full-length huntingtin accumulation in the cytoplasm, Neuron, 57(1):27-40.

30. Quarrell, O. (2008). Huntington's Diseas: The Facts (2nd ed) Oxford University Press, Oxford.

31. Stroke Association. (2009). What is a Stroke? www.stroke.org.uk Visited 02 03 09.

32. Stroke Help Association (2009). www.strokehelpassociation.org/ Visited 21 07 09.

33. Tarr M, BÜlthoff, H. (1995). Is Human Object Recognition Better Described By Geon Structural Descriptions Or Multiple Views? Comment On Biederman and Gerhardstein (1993) Journal of Experimental Psychology: Human Perception and Performance, 21, 1494-1505.

34. Vanacore, N. (2005). Epidemiological evidence on multiple system atrophy. Journal of Neural Transmission, 112(12):1605-12.

35. Van Dellen A, Blakemore C, Deacon R, York D, Hannan A.

(2000). Delaying the Onset of Huntington's in Mice Nature, 404, 721-722.

36. Wenning G, Colosimo C, Geser F. (2004). Mutliple System Atrophy, Lancet Neurology, 3:93-103.

Glossary

Alzheimer's Disease: The most common form of dementia. Many areas of the brain are affected, and there is a progressive loss of cognitive function including memory, perception and language.

Amygdala: A small almond shaped area (there are two, one in each hemisphere of the brain) that is part of the limbic system, and processes memory of emotional reactions.

Amyotrophic Lateral Sclerosis: Often referred to as Lou Gehrig's disease after the American basket ball player who had the condition. In France it is known as Charcot's disease (maladie de Charcot). It is one of the forms of motor neurone disease. There is progressive muscle wasting, spasticity and stiffness. It usually presents over the age of 50. Around 1 amongst 5 people survive more than 5 years, and there are examples of people living much longer.

Basal Nuclei: Dense areas of cells deep in the brain that connect with the cortex, the thalamus and the brain stem. They have many functions, and are particularly associated with motor control (organisation of movement) and learning.

Batik: An ancient art involving dying material and preserving the colour where it is wanted to be retained by applying hot wax, then drying, and then dying again. The process is repeated after preserving colour with the help of wax until the pre-conceived colour design is revealed as complete, after removing the wax protection. This is explained more fully in the section on complementary therapies under 'art therapy'.

Brain Stem: The base of the brain connecting with the spinal cord. It is made up of the medulla oblongata, the pons and the midbrain, and is important in regulating basic life functions such as heart rate and breathing.

Cerebrospinal Fluid: The fluid surrounding and protecting the brain and spinal cord.

Cerebal Palsy: An umberella term for a group of permanent, non-progressive disorders of the brain affecting movement and posture. There can be cognitive problems and other effects such as epilepsy, but often these don't occur. It is a congenital condition- meaning the damage to a brain leading to the disorder, occurs at or around the time of birth, or earlier in foetal development.

Cerebrum: The large part of the brain, divided into two hemispheres, with four lobes in each. It is what most people think of as 'the brain'.

Chorea: Uncoordinated dance-like involuntary movement.

Creutzfeld Jacob Disease: A rapid onset and deteriorating, progressive and fatal brain disorder. It is thought that the disease can be contracted by eating meat from animals with bovine disease, and it can be transmitted through growth hormone, corneal transplants and other invasive procedures.

Dementia: Cognitive decline resulting from brain degeneration, beyond what can be expected from normal aging. 'Mentia' refers to the mind, hence 'de-mentia' means detracted from the mind.

Dystonia: A movement disorder caused by neurological impairment, involving sustained muscle contractions, contorted posture and twisting, repetitive movements.

Episodic Memory: Episodes of the past experienced something like film clips.

Frontal Lobes: The front sections of each hemisphere in the brain (left and right). The frontal lobes are associated with higher thinking, planning and organising. They are involved in seeing things from another's point of view, and the ability to suppress impulses.

Huntington's Disease: A disorder of the brain leading to a movement disorder (notably chorea), cognitive decline, and psychiatric problems. The condition is eventually fatal although survival maybe anything from 8 to 30 or more years after the diagnosis. The onset of symptoms usually occurs in midlife, though there is a juvenile form. The condition is inherited as a dominant genetic trait. The offspring of those affected are at 50% risk of developing Huntington's.

Hypothalamus: An area above the brainstem important in regulating circadian rhythms (including waking and sleeping cycle), temperature and keeping many other body functions in balance.

Lewy Body Dementia: A form of dementia that is often, but not exclusively, associated with Parkinson's disease. The presentation varies but there tends to be a fluctuating condition with good, alert days, and days where cognition is poor. Hallucinations can occur- often perceiving the presence of a person appearing in the room. Reactions to drugs prescribed for conditions such as Alzheimer's disease can be life-threatening, and so differential diagnosis is crucial.

Meninges: The three protective layers (membranes) around the brain and spinal cord—the Pia mater (inner), arachnoid membrane, and the Dura mater (outer).

Motor Neurone Disease: (Or 'MND')- An umberella term for diseases in which motor neurones degenerate, affecting walking, speech, posture and breathing. There are four main types: Amyotrophic Lateral Sclerosis (ALS), Primary Lateral Sclerosis (PLS), Progressive Muscular Atrophy (PMA), and Bulbar MND which is divided into two types—Pseudobulbar Palsy and Progressive Bulbar Palsy. ALS affects both upper and lower motor neurones. PLS and pseudobulbar palsy affect upper motor neurones. PMA and progressive bulbar palsy affect lower motor neurones. Upper motor neurones carry motor signals from the brain down to the spinal cord, and lower motor neurones carry signals from the spinal cord to the muscles. Damage to upper neurones result in spasticity and brisk reflexes, whereas lower motor neurone damage leads to weak, flaccid muscles- muscle 'wasting'.

Multi-Infarct Dementia: A form of dementia resulting from a series of 'mini strokes', in which disruption to the flow of blood through the brain is caused by blockage of tiny blood vessels. This form is often referred to as 'vascular dementia'.

Multiple Sclerosis or 'disseminated sclerosis'-an auto-immune disease of the brain and spinal cord. 'Auto-immune' means that mechanisms in the person's immune system, normally working to protect the body, begin to attack part of the body, as though it were a harmful invader. In this case the myelin sheath around motor nerves, in multiple areas of the central nervous system is attacked. This impairs the transmission of signals from the brain to the muscles. Many people diagnosed with MS live a normal life with very little trouble from symptoms, such as tiredness or blurred vision. People who have 'Progressive MS' deteriorate steadily, and people with relapsing-remitting MS have spells of disability and spells of improvement.

Multiple System Atrophy: MSA is a progressive, degenerative neurological condition with symptoms including stiffness, muscle rigidity and slowness, tending to resemble those signs associated with Parkinson's disease. There are problems with balance and coordination and dizziness due to lowered blood pressure on standing up. There maybe many other symptoms and eventually due to swallowing difficulties, death frequently occurs through aspiration pneumonia (inhaling fluids over time) or choking. The condition is often misdiagnosed in the earlier stages.

Myoclonus: Sudden contractions of muscle groups. The sudden jerk many people have experienced at some time, just when dropping off to sleep, and hiccups are examples of myoclonus. In some individuals with some neurological disorders myoclonus can involve any groups of muscles, and can be very troublesome.

Occipital Lobe: The lobe at the back of each hemisphere of the brain, where vision is processed.

Parietal Lobe: The lobe in each hemisphere of the brain, above the occipital lobe and behind the frontal lobe. It is important in mapping out and making sense of the sensory information received by the brain, that is, in many aspects of perception, including visuo-spatial processing.

Parkinson's Disease: A progressive neurological condition characterised by a movement disorder, classically involving a resting tremor, slow movement and muscle rigidity. This 'shaking palsy' was described by James Parkinson in 1817.

Pick's Disease: A relatively rare, rapidly progressing neurological disease. Social skills deteriorate and there is impaired memory and intellect and personality change.

Procedural Memory: Long term memory of how to carry out skills that have been learned.

Progressive Bulbar Palsy: One of the forms of motor neurone disease, described under that heading, above.

Progressive Lateral Sclerosis: One of the forms of motor neurone disease, described under that heading, above.

Progressive Muscular Atrophy: One of the forms of motor neurone disease, described under that heading, above.

Spasticity: The continued tightening (contracting) of muscles due to neurological disorder.

Stroke: The sudden loss of oxygen supply in some part of the brain due to either a blockage in a blood vessel in the neck or the brain by a clot, usually of blood ('ischaemic stroke') or due to a haemorrhage (bleed) ('haemorrhagic stroke'). The consequences are potentially fatal. There is weakness on one side of the face and limbs, with slurred speech. The person maybe unconscious. With rapid treatment, the chances of survival and of avoiding lasting disability are greatly improved. Therefore, the public are advised to learn the 'FAST' response. Face - is one side drooping? Can the person smile? Arms - can the person raise both arms normally? Speech - is it slurred or impaired? Test - run the above test and if any of these problems are present, ring 999, and report a stroke... remember, Time is brain!!

Temporal Lobe: The lobes of the brain on each lower side of the cerebrum. If a boxing glove could represent the shape of the brain, loosely, the thumb would represent the temporal lobe's position. The temporal lobes process the meaning of language and visual information received. It overlies the hippocampus which is important in forming long term memories.

Thalamus: Seated in the midbrain, it relays sensory information coming in to the cortex, and relays motor information from the cortex. It is important in regulating consciousness.

Tics: Sudden non-rhythmic involuntary muscle movements.

Tourettes Syndrome: Tourretes is a spectrum of tic disorders, involving numerous motor muscle groups and causing involuntary vocal sounds. Some severe cases can be associated with unintended obscene or unpleasant remarks or exclamations, and the condition is better known for these rarer symptoms.

Transient Ischaemic Attack: A stroke (see 'Stroke' above) that resolves within 24 hours, leaving no residual effects. It should be reported as a medical emergency, as it is associated with a high risk of serious stroke.

Vascular Dementia: Dementia caused by problems with the delivery of blood to areas of the brain. The term 'vascular' refers to the vessels, in this case the tiny vessels that carry the blood, which brings oxygen to the brain. Dementia can result from a single stroke- known as 'single infarct dementia'. Dementia resulting from a series of 'mini-strokes' or damage to various parts of the tiny network of blood vessels in the brain is known as 'multi-infarct dementia'.

Visuo-spatial Awareness: The ability to map out the environment, and to understand and visualise objects and spatial relationships.

Working Memory: A theoretical concept relating to the way the brain organises and handles information stored briefly in short term memory.

Index